Cuisine, Colonialism and Cold War

CUISINE, COLONIALISM AND COLD WAR

FOOD IN TWENTIETH-CENTURY KOREA

Katarzyna J. Cwiertka

REAKTION BOOKS

To my mother

Published by Reaktion Books Ltd
33 Great Sutton Street
London EC1V 0DX, UK

www.reaktionbooks.co.uk

First published 2012

Printed and bound in Great Britain by
TJ International, Padstow, Cornwall

British Library Cataloguing in Publication Data
Cwiertka, Katarzyna Joanna, 1968–
Cuisine, colonialism and Cold War: food in twentieth-century Korea.
1. Food habits — Korea — History — 20th century.
2. Diet — Korea — History — 20th century.
3. Korea — Colonial influence.
4. Korea — Civilization — Japanese influences.
5. Cold War — Social aspects — Korea.
I. Title
394.1'2'09519'0904-DC23

ISBN 978 1 78023 025 2

Contents

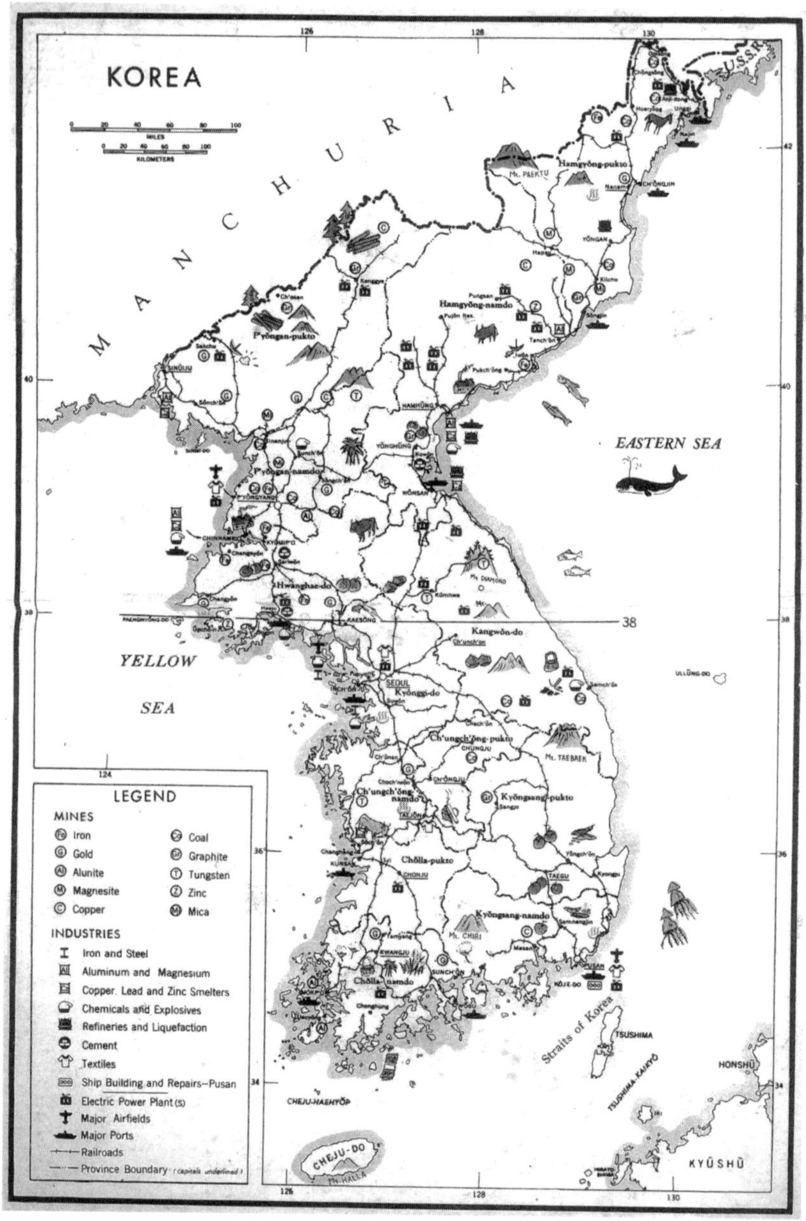

Map of Korea with its resources, early 1950s.

Introduction

> To many Westerners, the name Korea is apt to suggest far-flung battlefronts and cold wars rather than the unequivocal pleasures of the table. But the highly spiced, many-flavoured dishes of Korean cuisine are sure to become a memorable experience to anyone who has sampled them . . . Falling roughly between the remarkable diversity of Chinese cooking and the artistry of Japanese, Korean food has its own unique characteristics of spiced delectation. To go with the staple rice dish, a variety of soups and dishes are provided. The subtle flavours of the main courses are induced by careful additions of soy sauce, garlic, pepper, sesame seed, and other seasonings; these courses with subsidiary dishes will delight all lovers of good food.[1]

With these words the Charles E. Tuttle Company praises its publication *The Art of Korean Cooking* (1959), written by Harriett Morris, a Methodist missionary active in Korea and for many years the pillar of the Home Economics Department at Ewha Women's University in Seoul. The cookbook was published fifteen years after Ms Morris had returned to her home town of Wichita in Kansas, and six years after the ceasefire agreement put a halt to the hostilities of the Korean War (1950–53). The year 1959 fell in the heyday of the Cold War, just a few years before the Cuban Missile Crisis (October 1962) and the escalation of the Indochina conflict into a fully fledged Vietnam War (1965–75). It was around this time that Americans cautiously began to discover Asian food, with Korean and Japanese dishes still far less well known than the Chinese fare that had gained popularity during the 1940s.[2] Thai and

Vietnamese food were at this point totally absent from the American dining scene.

Precisely half a century later, the South Korean government launched an ambitious plan to turn Korean food into one of the five most popular 'ethnic' cuisines in the world (read 'in the United States') by 2017.[3] The objective is to situate Korean cuisine next to the Chinese, Thai, Vietnamese and Japanese foods that are nowadays immensely popular in North America.[4] Like other Asian governments, South Korean authorities have become conscious of the potential of food culture as a powerful ambassador of the Korean 'brand'.

The 50 years that passed between the publication of Morris's cookbook and the launch of the promotional campaign witnessed not only a shift on the American gastronomic scene, but a considerable transformation of the daily diet of the Korean population. Like elsewhere, a largely differentiated culinary landscape with rich regional and class variations was characteristic of the dietary culture of pre-modern Korea.[5] Food processing and preparation were a household affair, with recipes handed down from one generation to another. Today the food-processing industry and restaurant business are both thriving, and nutritional science has largely replaced the traditional concepts that had once guided food preparation and consumption. Ms Morris herself actively contributed to this process by teaching American home economics to Korean women in Seoul during the 1920s and '30s.

Before the twentieth century the pace of dietary change was slow on the Korean peninsula, with occasional innovations interrupting established patterns. The very foundation of Korean cuisine developed under the influence of the civilization of ancient China. This legacy is reflected, for example, in the use of chopsticks, the extensive consumption of processed soybeans (in soy sauce, soybean paste and soybean curd or tofu) and the position of rice as the preferred staple. It should be pointed out that rice had since ancient times been an exclusive ingredient not available to everyone on a daily basis. Millet, barley, sorghum, or rice combined with these grains or with beans, constituted the common fare of the majority of Koreans.[6] The old phrase 'white rice with meat soup' (*h'ŭin pap kwa kogiguk*), for example, connotes the image of the good life while tacitly acknowledging that not everyone could afford either rice or meat.

Because of the prominent place that grilled meat now occupies on the menus of Korean barbecue restaurants worldwide, Korean cuisine tends to be perceived as meat-focused, especially in comparison to

Thai, Vietnamese and Japanese cuisines, which are associated with vegetables and seafood. The taste for meat which is so pronounced in contemporary South Korea stands in strong contrast to the historically documented chronic shortage of meat in the daily Korean diet.[7] Before the economic growth of the 1970s, beef, pork, lamb, chicken and various types of game were only consumed regularly by the upper classes. Farmers, who before the twentieth century formed the majority of the Korean population, rarely ate meat except for three days in summer, when dog stew was served, and a special day in winter when sparrows, wild boar or wild rabbit were prepared. In both cases the eating of meat, which was not part of the daily diet, was intended to strengthen physical resistance against extreme weather conditions.[8]

Until a few decades ago, meat played a marginal role in Korean cooking, and it still remains a luxury in North Korea. The extensive consumption of vegetables qualifies much better as a distinctive and long-standing feature of Korean cuisine. There is a great variety of vegetable dishes – blanched, sautéed, pan-fried or pickled – and they still dominate practically every meal.

The Korean meal is structured around three components: boiled rice or other grain (*pap*), soup (*kuk* or *t'ang*) and pickled vegetables (*kimch'i*). Side dishes (*panch'an*) extend this core, and their number depends

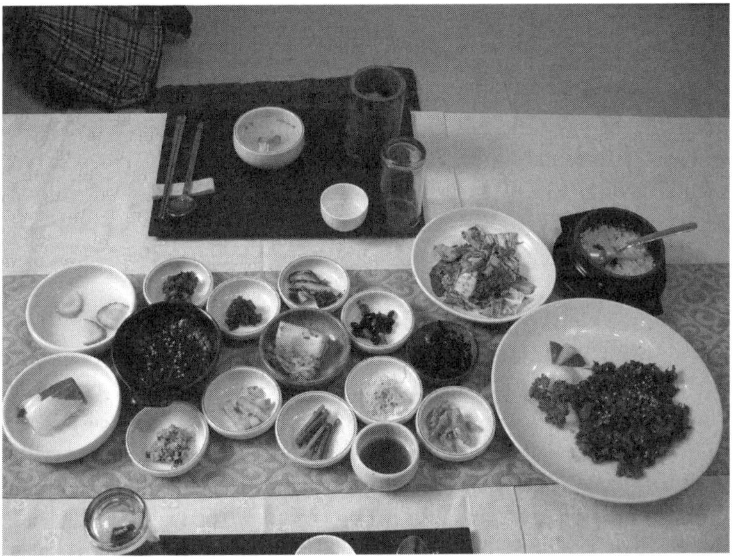

A Korean meal served at an upmarket restaurant in Seoul, 2003.

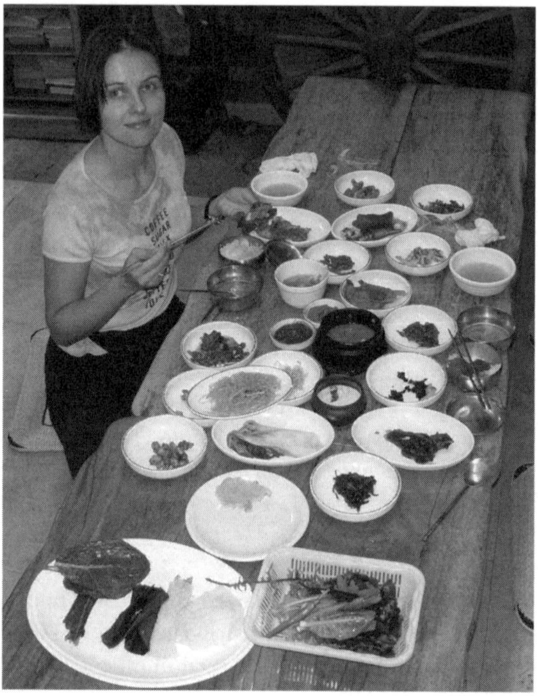

The author enjoying an overwhelmingly vegetarian Korean meal, 2003.

on the occasion and economic status of the diners. It is the norm to serve between three and five side dishes at daily meals in contemporary South Korean households, but this number would have been considered a luxury in the past, and this is still the case in North Korea today. Stews and soused or sautéed greens are the most common side dishes, complemented by more lavish grilled and braised food prepared with seafood, beef, pork or chicken. Stews and grilled dishes tend to acquire the position of a semi-main dish, becoming the centre of the meal, accompanied by a bowl of rice, soup and smaller side dishes.

Three kinds of fermented soybean condiments – soy sauce (*kanjang*), soybean paste (*toenjang*) and hot red chilli paste (*koch'ujang*) – along with chillies, sesame (seed and oil), garlic and spring onions constitute what might be called a 'Korean flavour'. The combination of all or a selection of these ingredients gives Korean dishes their characteristic taste. The technology of soybean fermentation was introduced from China during Korea's Three Kingdoms period (57 BC–AD 668), gradually leading to the development of liquid soy sauce and solid soybean paste. Hot red chilli paste, the third and perhaps most distinctive condiment

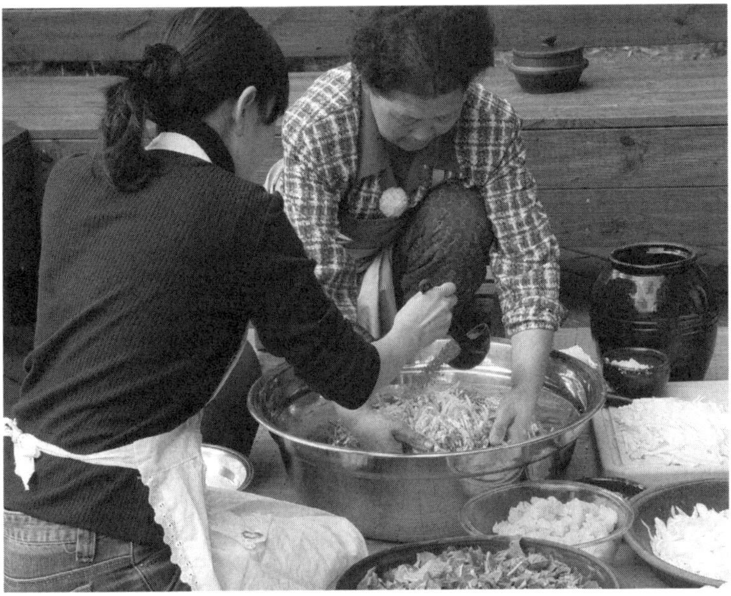

Chilli powder being added during the preparation of *kimch'i*, 2003.

in the Korean soybean trinity, emerged several centuries later following the introduction of the chilli. This New World plant entered Korea via Japan around the turn of the fifteenth and the sixteenth century.[9]

The incorporation of the chilli into Korean cuisine is perhaps the most revolutionary innovation in its pre-modern history. As well as the development of hot red chilli paste, chillies fundamentally transformed the taste and appearance of the most basic, indispensable element of every Korean meal, *kimch'i* pickle, without which neither a feast nor the most meagre fare would be complete. The process of pickling vegetables, generally referred to by this name, was considerably transformed between the seventeenth and the nineteenth century.[10] Besides adding chillies and reducing the use of salt, an important modification was the introduction in the mid-nineteenth century of the practice of seasoning *kimch'i* with fermented seafood (*chŏtkal*). This innovation not only enriched the taste of *kimch'i* but greatly enhanced its regional diversity, expanding the number of varieties to over 200, as each locality pickled different kinds of seafood according to slightly different procedures. Yet it is the chilli that gives *kimch'i* its distinctive red colour and pungent taste. With its reddishness and spiciness, *kimch'i* functions as the most powerful icon of Korean cuisine. It is also emblematic of the South Korean hegemony over the image of Korean cuisine, since North Korean varieties of the pickle utilize chillies much more sparingly.

The pace of change on the Korean peninsula – including dietary developments – was greatly accelerated after the turn of the twentieth century by two sweeping forces of history: colonialism and war. Korea's encounter with the former began in the late nineteenth century when the peninsula became the scene for a power struggle between the Chinese, Japanese and Russian empires. At this point, the influence of China on Korea's historical development had already been strong and long-standing. In contrast, the growing involvement of Japan in the affairs of its neighbour was not only new but devastating. On 29 August 1910 Korea fell under Japanese colonial rule, which lasted for 35 years and ended officially on 2 September 1945 with the signing of the Instruments of Surrender, a formal document that followed the announcement of Japan's capitulation eighteen days earlier.

Half a century after becoming the central stage for a power struggle between the colonial powers in Asia, Korea yet again gained the attention of international politics as the first theatre of the Cold War. While the legacies of Cold War in Germany and Vietnam have been successfully resolved since the fall of the Berlin Wall in 1989, the 38th parallel still divides the northern and southern half of the Korean peninsula. It is a vivid reminder that Korea remains the only place in the world where the Cold War never ended.

Historians of modern Korea have argued that the country has played a disproportionately important role in the last 100 years of the world's history in relation to the size of its population and breadth of its territory.[11] By turning this statement around, one could claim that world history has played a disproportionately important role in twentieth-century Korea. This is precisely the intention of this volume. By using food as the focus of analysis, I seek to demonstrate that the lives of contemporary Koreans, both in the North and in the South, have been largely shaped by colonialism and Cold War.

Being forced from the margins to the centre of the world system, the peninsula experienced colonial submission, occupation, war, violent social upheavals and ongoing national division. The ambition of this book is to pin down these events as they were echoed in the mundane details of cuisine. Chapter One describes Korea as the breadbasket of the Japanese Empire after its annexation as a colony in 1910. Chapter Two portrays the introduction of new modes of consumption in the colonial cities, and chapter Three focuses on the legacy of Japanese colonialism in the industrialization of soy sauce manufacture that has led to the homogenization of the flavour of Korean dishes. Chapter Four examines dietary conditions during the Sino-Japanese War (1937–45) and the Korean War (1950–53), while chapters Five and Six shed light on the developments in North and South Korea after the armistice of 1953.

The recent global promotion of Korean cuisine by the South Korean government stands in contrast with the hunger and malnutrition still prevailing in North Korea. The rock bottom of the crisis took place between 1994 and 1999, but the dire food situation continues to the present day. This tragic episode ends the odyssey of twentieth-century Korea as depicted through the lens of food. The book concludes with remarks on Korean food at the dawn of the twenty-first century and general observations on culinary nostalgia and the commodification of tradition.

Wherever possible I refer to English-language rather than Korean- and Japanese-language sources. All Korean and Japanese terms throughout this book have been indicated in italics, except for personal, geographical and institutional names. Korean terms are romanized according to the McCune-Reischauer system and Japanese terms according to the Hepburn system of romanization, with the exception of widely used geographical names, such as Seoul, Pyongyang, Tokyo, Osaka and the four largest Japanese islands. In cases where a specific name romanization is preferred by an organization or an individual, it will be applied here as well. Korean and Japanese names are given in the traditional East Asian order with the surname first, except for the authors of English-language publications. When referring to Korean geographical names during the colonial period, I use their Korean names, except for the colonial capital of Keijō (present-day Seoul) and its street and districts. The above principles are not applied to quotations, where the formats of the original source are retained. When referring to the Republic of Korea (ROK) and the Democratic People's Republic of Korea (DPRK), I will alternate between these official names and the commonly used 'South Korea' and 'North Korea'.

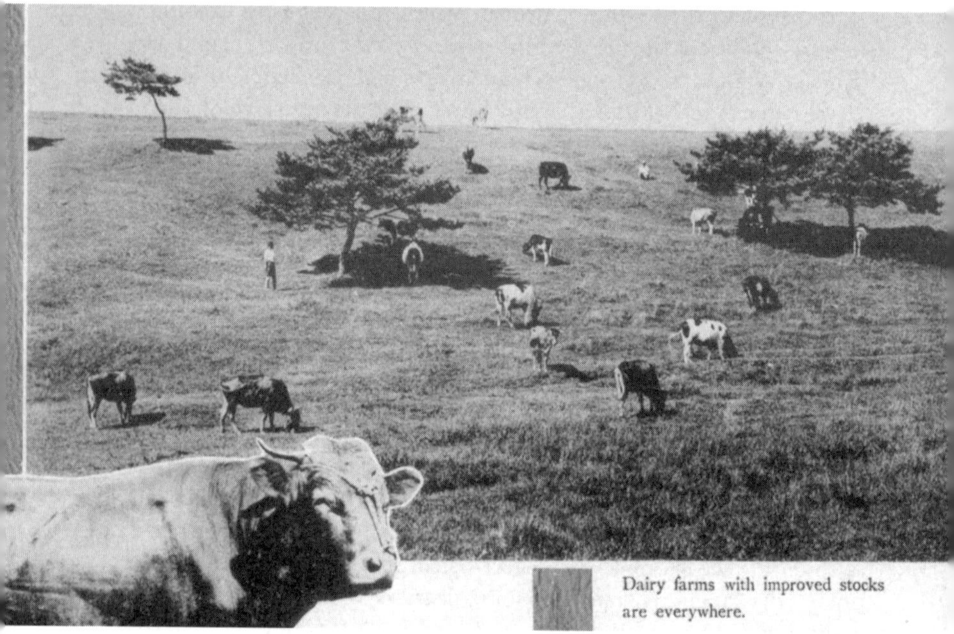

In the early twentieth century, animal husbandry was envisaged as an important area of growth for the Korean economy.

1
Breadbasket of the Japanese Empire

Japanese Imperialism in Korea

Korea entered the twentieth century in a politically unstable condition. Since the Kanghwa Treaty of 1876, when the country was forced to establish commercial and diplomatic relations with the outside world, its sovereignty had been gradually compromised until it finally became the victim of Japanese colonialism. The rivalry between China and Japan over influence on the peninsula culminated in the First Sino-Japanese War (1894–5), which marked the ascendance of Japan – at the time a novice in Western-dominated global politics – to the status of a regional power. The fate of Korea was finally sealed ten years later following Japan's victory in a war with Russia, another rival in the scramble for the peninsula. The conditions of the Treaty of Portsmouth, which formally ended the Russo-Japanese War (1904–5) and set the balance of power in the Pacific for decades to come, gave Japan the right to control Korea. During the first five years this control took the form of a 'protectorate', which in practice meant that the Korean government had to cede control of its foreign affairs to Japan. In the summer of 1910 Korea finally became incorporated into the Japanese Empire as its colony.

Exploring any aspect of Japanese colonialism in Korea is contentious, and this period of Korean history tends to become heavily loaded with ideological implications and political sentiments. On the one hand, the claims by Japanese colonialists that they were modernizing Asia and the use of these claims to justify colonial rule are still remembered vividly among the colonized peoples, and resurface even today in the activities of revisionist groups.[1] On the other, the politicization of the historical record in the Democratic People's Republic of Korea (North Korea) and the Republic of Korea (South Korea) created favourable circumstances for the longstanding domination of a homogenized view of Japanese colonialism as repression and exploitation. A clear-cut picture of the Japanese as aggressors and the Koreans as patriots still dominates the public discourse on the colonial period in many respects. Yet the 35 years of Japanese rule are too complex to be simply labelled as 'colonial exploitation'.

The Japanese colonial period (1910–45) was for Korea a time of complicated and ambivalent historical processes in which colonialism, modernity and identity were mutually constitutive.[2] The loss of sovereignty and the colonial experience, for example, played a critical role in the rise of Korean nationalism.[3] While eagerly exploiting Korea's resources for its own goals, Japan also provided a blueprint for Korea's industrialization, functioning in many respects as a mentor in the lesson of how to modernize following the Western model. More than three decades of colonial rule transformed the country in practically every respect: its transportation and administrative networks, financial and commercial structures, education system and gender and labour relations, as well as leisure and consumption practices. A peculiar feature of those transformations was their association with the colonizer, since they were largely shaped by the agenda of the Japanese authorities and enterprises, and often utilized templates that had been developed in Japan – based on Western models – decades earlier in the process of its own modernization. To be modern in colonial Korea inevitably entailed association with Japanese rule, forcing the colonized to adopt the colonizers' language and values, or at least required tacit acceptance of the colonial culture.[4] Such ambiguous processes lay at the root of twentieth-century Korea.

While Japanese propaganda heralded the civilizing aspects of Korea's colonization, it would be naive to assume that various projects undertaken by the Japanese in order to modernize – and at a later stage industrialize – the colony were carried out for the sake of the Korean people. Japanese rule in Korea was fully and foremost 'in the furtherance of Japanese interests'.[5] That the reforms instigated by the colonial authorities and Japanese entrepreneurs also served as the groundwork of Korea's modernization was merely a by-product, never an objective, of the colonizing project.

The colony was ruled by the Japanese Governor-General of Korea (Chōsen Sōtokufu), who was appointed directly by the Japanese emperor and operated with absolute authority and considerable autonomy. While in Japan different administrative functions – such as authority over the police, legislative bodies, and judicial and fiscal systems – belonged to separate ministries, in Korea they were all concentrated in the person of the Governor-General. Although highly centralized, the system penetrated into every corner of the colony. By directly appointing the chief officials of provinces, counties, cities and townships, the office of the Governor-General extended strict control over local affairs. This took place through an extensive administrative apparatus of Japanese administrators which in time was supplemented by Koreans who had been educated through the newly instituted Japanese-style education system. By 1937, 52,270 Japanese and 35,282 Koreans were employed by the colonial bureaucracy.[6]

Replicating the relationship between the Western empires and their colonies worldwide, Korea was envisaged by the Japanese colonial authorities as a breadbasket of the Empire and a consumer market for Japanese manufactured products. Efficient exploitation of Korean agricultural resources was to be achieved in the first place through the promotion of modern agricultural technology. Technological transfer was supported by the colonial government, guided by agricultural specialists from Japan, and facilitated through local administrative organizations, often with the aid of the police.[7] The first steps were taken soon after the establishing of Japan's protectorate in 1905, and steadily accelerated with the annexation. In 1906, for example, the first agricultural experimental station was set up and the Korea Central Agricultural Association, the precursor of the Korean Farmers' Association, was established. In 1908 two experimental seeding stations were established: one in South Kyŏngsang Province, in the southeastern tip of the peninsula closest to Japan, and one in South Ch'ungch'ŏng Province, south of the colonial capital of Keijō. Five more such stations were set up in other provinces over the next two years and a decade later some of them began to publish reports that disseminated information on various diseases that could affect various crops and how to deal with them. In March 1912 an Agricultural Technology Bureau (Nōgyō Gijutsukan) was established in every province; these were to become responsible for planning the development of animal husbandry and the production of silk, cotton and rice.[8]

Following the Japanese penetration of Manchuria after 1931, the role of Korea within the Japanese Empire began to shift from peacetime breadbasket to military stockroom. Korea was to be industrialized in order to exploit the raw materials of neighbouring Manchuria. Japan's withdrawal from the League of Nations in 1933, in response to the League's criticism of Japan's invasion of this northeastern Chinese

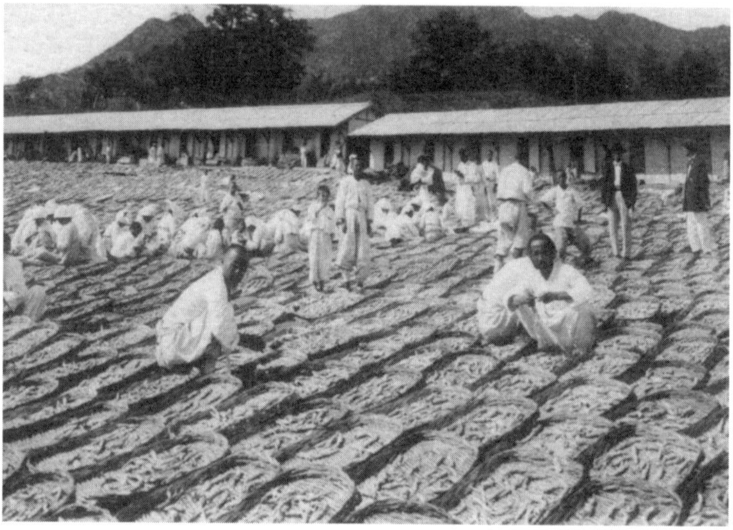

Breadbasket of the Empire: ginseng, *c.* 1920s.

territory, clearly demonstrated that the country was determined to intensify its military encroachment into the Asian continent. The outbreak of the Second Sino-Japanese War in 1937 and the attack on the Philippines and Pearl Harbor in 1941 transformed Japan into a total-war empire that geared all its colonies towards wartime mobilization. For Korea, these circumstances translated into rapid industrial development.

The remarkable industrialization of the colony during the 1930s and early '40s is generally associated with the growth of mining and heavy industry through the investments of large Japanese business combines known as *zaibatsu*, including Mitsubishi, Nissan, Sumitomo and Nitchitsu.[9] However, this period was also crucial for the development of industrial food processing in Korea. Modern, state-of-the-art factories were set up to secure a supply line for provisioning Japanese armed forces encroaching into the Asian continent. By the 1930s beer, ship's biscuits and canned food constituted the mainstays of the diet of the Japanese military.[10]

Rice functions as a very powerful symbol of Japanese colonialism in Korea. The deprivation of the Korean population of its staple food while ever-increasing quantities were exported to feed Japanese urban consumers virtually stands for the colonial exploitation of Korea.[11] As this chapter will demonstrate, however, the story of Korea as the breadbasket of the Japanese Empire is far more complex. Besides rice,

Korea's other food resources and the industry that was developed to process them played a critical role in sustaining Japan's military expansion into Asia.

Rice

The 1890s marked a turning point in Japan's economic development that is characteristic of the transition from an agricultural to an industrial economy. A long phase of mutually reinforcing growth in agriculture and manufacturing came to an end, and Japan experienced for the first time the constraints on industrial development caused by inadequate growth in the domestic food supply.[12] Only a decade earlier, the growth in the consumption of rice had still barely matched the growth in output, so exports were promoted by the government as a means to earn foreign exchange. However, the bad harvest of 1889–90 put an end to this new strategy, resulting instead in the opening of Japan for rice imports. Within only one decade (between 1883–7 and 1893–7), the share of imports in the total amount of rice consumed skyrocketed from 0.1 to 2.59 per cent, reaching nearly 10 per cent ten years later.[13]

At first the bulk of rice imports came from Southeast Asia, in particular the regional 'rice bowls' of the Irrawaddy Delta in Burma, the Chao Phraya Delta in Siam and the Mekong Delta in Cochin China. These three areas accounted for approximately 90 per cent of the rice entering the world export market between 1910 and 1935.[14] In the early years of the twentieth century the quantities of Korean rice exported to Japan were relatively small, and up to the 1920s no measures towards increasing these exports were undertaken, mainly due to the interests of Japanese landlords, who lobbied for the maintenance of the stable, high price of rice.[15] It is quite plausible that this policy would have continued were it not for the developments following the outbreak of the First World War in 1914. The implementation of export restrictions on Southeast Asian rice by the British and French colonial authorities following the outbreak of the First World War provided the first incentive for structural changes in the pattern of rice imports in Japan. The restrictions created a severe rice shortage in major Japanese cities, driving prices up and leading in 1918 to the so-called Rice Riots (*kome sōdō*). The riots served as a direct stimulus for the Japanese government to adopt a policy specifying that the Empire should be self-sufficient in food. This goal was achieved by the 1930s, with the colonies of Taiwan and Korea supplying 95–8 per cent of Japanese rice imports.[16]

The impact of the Rice Riots proved particularly powerful due to the international context of the time. Japanese policymakers, who had carefully observed the situation in Europe, were particularly struck by the collapse of the German Empire and the close connection of this downfall with the inability to secure food resources. Isolated riots over the quickly deteriorating food situation had begun to take place in larger German towns in 1915. Food shortages inflicted by the Allied blockade and successive bad harvests, in conjunction with the hesitant and unsystematic approach of German authorities to food management, had ultimately led to the November Revolution of 1918 and to Germany's defeat.[17] This experience seems to have left a lasting impression on Adolf Hitler. In September 1939, just before embarking on his war, Germany was equipped with stocks of raw materials and a grain reserve of 6 million tonnes, which could compensate for the import requirements of approximately three years.[18] The policymakers in Japan drew the same conclusion, turning food autarky within the Empire into a top priority and Korea into its rice granary. Between 1915–19 and 1935–9 the export of Korean rice to Japan multiplied 3.8 times from 15 to 37 per cent of the total output of Korean agriculture.[19] This increase is even more spectacular when we consider that

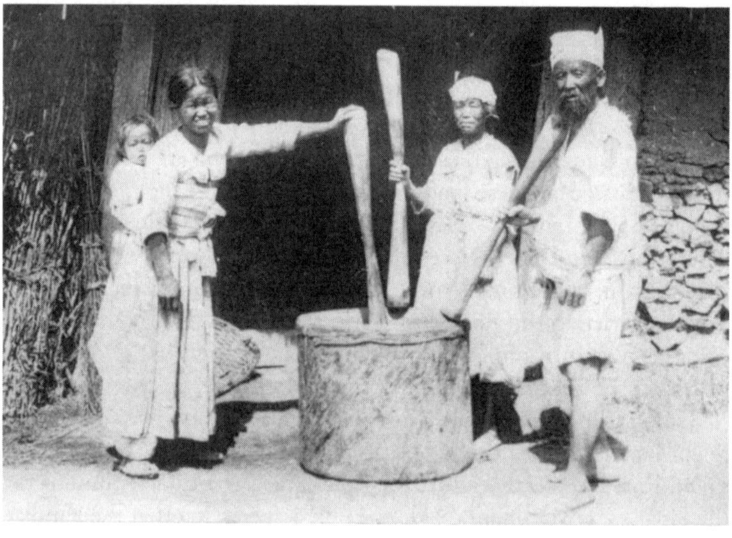

Korean farmers polishing rice, *c.* 1910s.

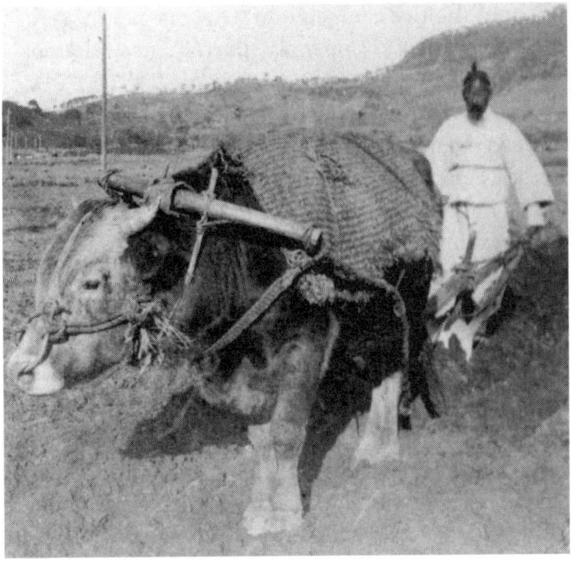

A Korean farmer ploughing a field with an ox, c. 1901.

the volume of rice production in Korea during this period increased by more than 250 per cent.[20]

This massive increase was possible in the first place due to an improvement of farming methods; the amount of land under cultivation increased by merely 5 per cent throughout the aforementioned period.[21] The systematic introduction and dissemination of new technology, such as high-yield seed varieties, better irrigation systems and the use of commercial fertilizers, was carried out under the auspices of the Campaign to Increase Rice Production (*Sanmai zōshoku keikaku*), which was launched in 1920. The campaign also called for the reclamation and improvement of 800,000 hectares of paddy land over 30 years through controlled irrigation. However, these ambitious plans were never to be realized. After the initial phase (1920–25) the campaign was discontinued due to a shortage of funds. The second phase began in 1926 when a new source of funding was secured but was called off eight years later, when the government decided to abandon the programmes for increasing rice production in the colonies in the hope that slower agricultural growth would help to improve conditions in rural Japan.[22] The importation of inexpensive rice from the colonies was in fact threatening the livelihood of Japanese farmers and caused discontent in rural Japan. Moreover, investment in the industrialization of Korea began to acquire priority over agriculture from the 1930s onwards. The third phase of the rice campaign in Korea began in 1940, along with other measures that the Imperial Government undertook in order to fight the wartime food shortage.

The main reason why rice acquired the status of symbol of colonial exploitation is the fact that the massive increase in exports of Korean rice to Japan did not come about through increased rice production alone, but also entailed a quantitative sacrifice of the level of food consumption among the Korean population. Between 1911–12 and 1937–8, the exportation of rice reduced the annual per capita availability of rice for consumption in Korea from about 100 kg to 75 kg, enabling Japan to maintain its annual per capita consumption of rice at about 160 kg.[23] The period of greatest curtailment fell between 1932 and 1936, when barley, millet and wheat were imported to Korea from Manchuria in order to substitute for the shortage of rice.[24] Since the volume of imported grain was not sufficient to balance the deficit, the increasing rice exports involved not only a qualitative sacrifice in substituting coarse grains for rice, but also a quantitative sacrifice in terms of food consumed.[25]

It is beyond dispute that the Japanese strategy of ensuring the self-sufficiency of its Empire in terms of food supply created a heavy burden for the Korean population. In the long run, Korean rice allowed Japan to save foreign exchange that would otherwise have had to be spent on rice imports from Southeast Asia. The shift from 'foreign' to

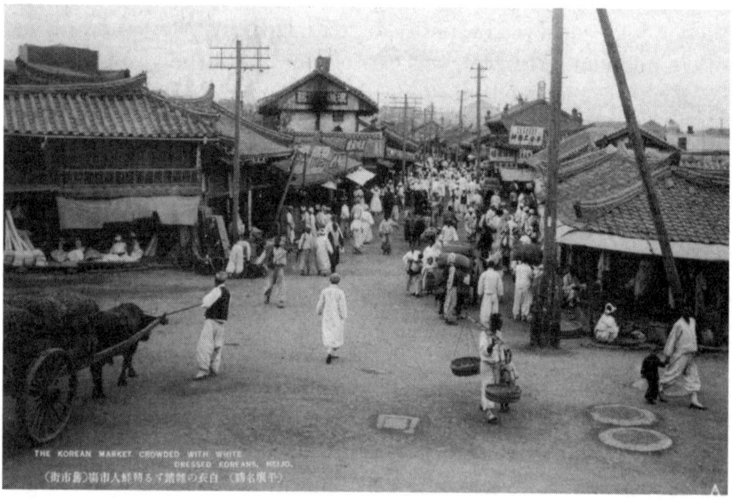

A market in Heijō (today's Pyongyang), *c.* 1930s.

'colonial' rice to secure the demand of the growing urban population thus facilitated Japan's further industrialization by helping to keep the industrial wage low. As economic historians explain, however, this was a mixed blessing, since cheap colonial rice contributed to the ailing of the Japanese rural economy, which in turn provided the springboard for military reformists to effect military expansion on the Asian continent and ultimately led to the fall of the Empire.[26]

Food Processing

The symbolism of rice as an emblem of colonial exploitation, and its significant role in the strategies of empire, distracts our attention from other instances of utilization of Korean food resources by the Japanese. Food processing provides a perfect starting point from which to draw a picture of the transformation the colony underwent in order to meet the needs of Japan's rising militarist ambitions.

Before the mid-1930s, when mining and other branches of heavy industry began to emerge, the country was an agricultural economy with a highly underdeveloped manufacturing sector. During the first decade of colonial rule, which was known under the name Military Rule (*budan seiji*) and infamous for excessive repression of public life, industrial development was effectively discouraged. The so-called Korean Company Law (Chōsen Kaisha Rei) issued immediately after Korea's annexation required new companies to be officially licensed by the Government-General, and subsidiaries or branch offices of foreign enterprises were plainly unwelcome.[27] From the 1920s onwards, with the shift towards a more liberal colonial administration known as Cultural Rule (*bunka seiji*), political and economic changes created new opportunities for Korea's industrialization. As agriculture was the key economic asset of the peninsula, it is not surprising that food processing became the first sector of the Korean industry to develop, and remained the major industrial activity throughout the colonial period.

Between 1922 and 1933, the number of food-processing companies operating in Korea increased fourfold, from approximately 500 to over 2,000.[28] By 1939 Korea had 2,399 food-processing factories generating production worth 447,595,991 yen, which constituted 39 per cent of the gross value of total industrial production in Korea.[29] In terms of value, the food-processing sector was still the largest, although its share had diminished by 25 per cent compared to six years earlier.[30]

The majority of food-processing factories in colonial Korea were relatively small and classified as 'household industry', implying that production was conducted at the home of the entrepreneur by members of his family, and in most cases simply constituted a subsidiary occupation of the farming population.[31] Most factories relied upon traditional production methods and required neither advanced technology nor high investments. Statistically, these primitive forms of manufacturing prevailed. However, modern, large-scale enterprises which employed more than 200 workers also operated, and their share steadily increased during the 1930s. For example, between 1933 and 1939, the number of food-processing factories which employed more than 50 workers increased from 6 to 76, those employing 100–200 workers from 4 to 40, and those employing more than 200 workers from 3 to 12.[32]

The overwhelming majority (nearly three-quarters) of food-processing factories in colonial Korea were rice-cleaning and rice-polishing mills and alcohol distilleries, but a wide variety of other food-processing enterprises were represented as well. In 1933 the three largest food-processing ventures were Japan Grain Industries (Nihon Kokusan Kōgyō) in Pyongyang, established by the Mitsubishi concern in 1931, Kurasawa Crab Cannery (Kurasawa Kanzume Kōjō), set up in 1923 on the shore of South Hamgyŏng Prefecture, and Katō Rice Mill (Katō Seimaijo), which had operated in Inch'ŏn since 1920.[33] Six years later, the largest factories were involved in rice cleaning and polishing (Pusan, Kunsan, two in Inch'ŏn and two in South P'yŏngan Prefecture); marine processing (two in South Hamgyŏng and one in North Hamgyŏng Prefecture); beef canning (South Hamgyŏng Prefecture); confectionery production (Pusan); and grain processing (Pyongyang).[34] The majority of medium-sized factories were rice-cleaning and rice-polishing enterprises (nineteen), canneries (nine), alcohol and soy sauce breweries (six), confectioners (three) and dried fish manufacturers (three).

A noteworthy development that took place during the 1930s was the slow yet steady growth in Korea of the manufacturing of Westernized products such as soft drinks, beer, bread and Western-style confectionery. Production grew in the first place to meet the increasing demand generated by the growing number of Japanese expatriates who had migrated to Korea (see chapter Two) rather than being due to the rising popularity of these products among the Korean population. Such products were imported into the colony at first. The Japanese upmarket Western-style grocer Meidi-ya had opened a sales branch in Seoul in 1908, mainly in order to expand the sales of Kirin beer, for which it held exclusive selling rights at the time. Next to beer, the store sold wines and liquors, biscuits, chocolate and a variety of other kinds of imported Western food and drink.[35] But by the 1930s local manufacturers were competing with the imports. Keijō confectioners – Tōa Seika, Chōsen Seika, Nagaoka Seika, Ōnari Seika and Keijō Kashi – each employing 100 or more workers, were involved in the large-scale production of chocolate, caramel and biscuits.[36]

By the late 1930s the products made by these pioneering manufacturers of Western-style food and drink in Korea were also increasingly consumed by Koreans. Beer and carbonated drinks, bread and Western-style confectionery, which were cheaper than imports from Japan, gradually acquired a niche in the consumption practices of the urban population, often functioning as symbols of modern life. Some products even began to function as local specialities, as was the case with cider and other bubble drinks from Ch'ŏngju, Taejŏn pound cake (*k'asŭt'ella*) and walnut cakes (*hodu kwaja*) from Ch'ŏnan.[37]

The manufacture of Western-style confectionery and drinks was conducted exclusively by Japanese entrepreneurs, often by setting up colonial branches of ventures that were already successfully operating in Japan. For example, in 1936 the colonial capital of Keijō had six soft drink manufacturers, six bakers, a chewing-gum factory and several pastry shops, including a branch of the famous Fujiya in Tokyo.[38] After 1932, when Japan formally established its rule over Manchuria through the puppet-state of Manchukuo, expanding Japanese enterprises into Korea entailed additional business opportunities offered by the proximity of Manchuria. The leading Japanese wheat flour producer, Nisshin Seifun, is a prime example of such expansion strategies.

The growing production of bread, biscuits and pastry in Korea generated a rising demand for wheat flour, which in turn had to be imported from Japan. In 1936, anticipating the growing opportunity for profit, Nisshin Seifun began to expand into Korea. Its subsidiary, Chōsen Seifun Company, operated three wheat-flour milling factories in the colony: the first one opened in Keijō in May 1937, followed by a second in Chinnampo in March 1939 and the last one in Haeju in January 1941 (the latter two located in the northern part of the peninsula). As the wheat supply deteriorated, the factories expanded their operations and began to mill maize, buckwheat and sorghum, as well as processing soybean cakes. A subsidiary of Chōsen Seifun – Oriental

Yeast Industry (Tōyō Kōbo Kōgyō), set up in 1941 – supplied bakeries, breweries and alcohol manufacturers with fermentation starters.[39]

The strategic locations of the Chōsen Seifun factories remind us that Japanese food-processing enterprises not infrequently set up factories in Korea not only with the civilian market in mind, but in anticipation of orders from the Japanese armed forces which were encroaching into the Asian continent. The leading Japanese confectionery producer Morinaga opened a factory in Keijō in 1940 and two years later enlarged the premises. Next to candies and biscuits for the civilian market, the factory produced portable rations for the army and air squadrons.[40] Another major Japanese confectionery firm, Meiji Seika, set up a factory in Keijō in 1943 to fulfil military orders for hardtack.[41]

A relatively early example of the successful expansion of the Japanese food-processing industry into Korea is that of the leading Japanese brewers Dai Nippon Beer Company and Kirin Beer Company, which almost simultaneously launched production in Korea in the early 1930s. The former established the Chōsen Beer Company in August 1933, and in December of the same year the latter set up Shōwa Kirin Beer Company. The beer produced in colonial Korea was largely consumed on the peninsula, in the late 1930s primarily by the Japanese armed forces.[42] Unlike biscuits, only a small share of Korean beer production was shipped overseas, as beer bottles were heavy and broke easily. Instead, both Dai Nippon Beer Company and Kirin Beer Company expanded their operations throughout Asia to supply the Japanese soldiers. They jointly operated the Manchuria Beer Company with two breweries in Mukden, one producing the Sapporo brand beer and the other the Kirin brand.[43] Following the expansion of the Japanese Empire southwards in 1941 and 1942, these two firms also became involved in managing breweries in the captured territories. For example, on the request of the Japanese army, Dai Nippon took up the operation of one brewery in each of Shanghai and Singapore and two in Manila. Kirin managed the Malayan Brewery in Singapore and two breweries in the Dutch East Indies: Archipel Brewery in Batavia and a subsidiary of Heineken Brewery in Surabaya.[44]

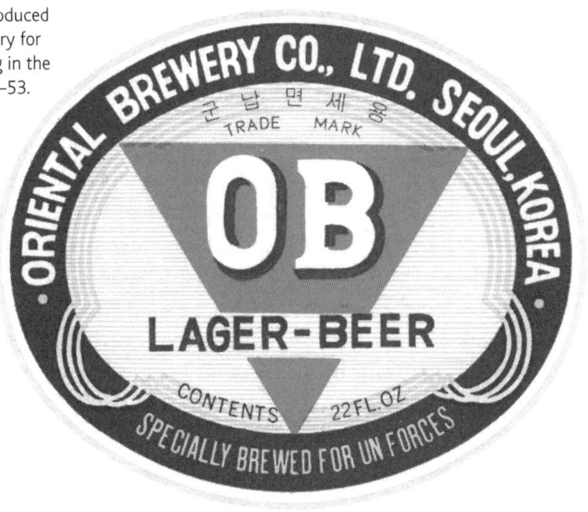

Label of a beer produced by Oriental Brewery for UN forces fighting in the Korean War, 1950–53.

Beef and Sardines

The sterilization and vacuum sealing of food, which later came to be widely known under the name of 'canning', are regarded along with refrigeration as the two pillars of industrial cuisine.[45] The 'discovery' of this method is attributed to the Parisian confectioner Nicolas Appert (1749–1841), who in 1809 was the first to succeed in demonstrating that it was possible to preserve food with this method. The next step in the history of the canning industry was taken the following year when the Englishman Peter Durand replaced Appert's glass containers with vessels made of tinplate.[46] The latter proved so much better suited for the purpose that they were soon utilized to supply sea voyagers, explorers, armed forces and expatriate Western communities in remote corners of the world with preserved food that they were not able to acquire in a fresh form.[47]

Warfare has from the very outset played a prominent role in the development of the canning industry. The method of Nicolas Appert, on which the modern industry depends, was developed on the basis of earlier practices and devices in response to an appeal from the French government for solutions in providing the army with food that had a long life and was easy to transport.[48] War continued to propel the production as well as the consumption of canned food in various times and locations: the American Civil War provided an enormous boost for the rise of the canning industry in the United States and the First

World War opened up the civilian market for canned food in France.[49] Imperialism constituted the second major force that shaped the canning industry. Canned food not only made it possible for expatriate communities to retain their distinctive food patterns, and protected them from the potential danger of contagion through food, but also carried with it an aura of modernity and superiority.[50] As canned food could be eaten out of season and out of place, and securely transported over great distances, canning technology also made a serious contribution to the strength of the Western armies and navies and therefore indirectly fostered Western territorial expansion.

When the newly formed Japanese government embarked in the early 1870s on its ambitious mission of 'catching up with the West' by enthusiastically importing Western technology and institutions, canning was not left unnoticed. Two reasons stood behind the governmental support for the canning industry. First, the strong orientation of the new government towards industrialization placed canning alongside the telegraph, the railway and other technological innovations as an emblem of progress and modernity. The second reason was related to the Japanese trade imbalance. As the investment required for setting up a canning business was minimal and the Japanese population was overwhelmingly agrarian, the authorities hoped that canning would soon flourish in Japan and that canned products would join rice, tea and raw silk as Japanese exports. It took several decades, however, before Japanese cans were able to meet these expectations and compete with American and European products on the global market. In the meantime, the infant industry was sustained largely by orders from the Japanese armed forces.[51] The First Sino-Japanese War (1894–5) and the Russo-Japanese War (1904–5), which provided an enormous stimulus for the Japanese canning industry, also facilitated the exploitation of Korean beef.

Korean cattle were exported to Japan decades before Korean rice assumed significance in the food strategies of the Japanese colonial empire. However, the Russo-Japanese War brought about a spectacular increase in the demand for Korean beef. The volume of exports increased from approximately 100 head of Korean cattle per annum during the 1880s and 1890s to nearly 20,000 Korean cows being transported to Japan in 1907 to be processed into canned-meat provisions supplied to the Imperial Japanese Army and Navy. Ironically the Japanese victory in that war led directly to the loss of Korea's independence.[52]

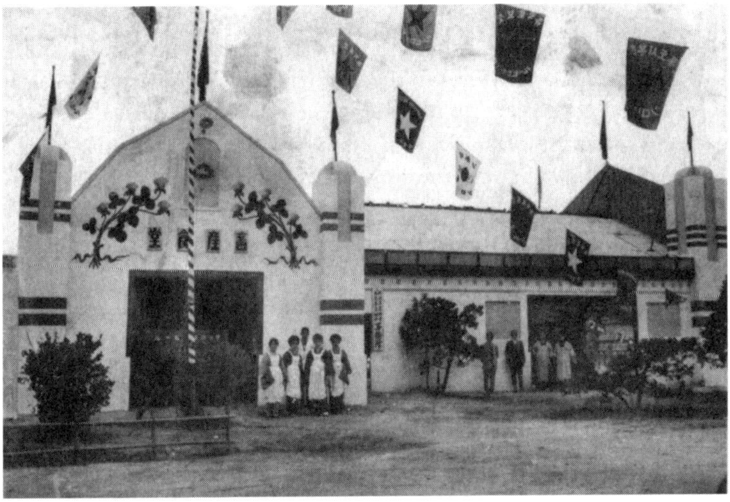

An eatery run by the Korea Animal Husbandry Association (Chōsen Chikusan Kyōkai), *c.* 1920s.

Stimulating the Korean beef industry became a priority of the colonial authorities early on. Following the annexation of 1910 the stock of Korean cattle increased by approximately 200,000 head per annum, by the 1920s exceeding 1.5 million head.[53] A steady supply of cheap Korean beef enabled the Japanese urban masses to embrace the culinary modernity represented by the Western-style dishes served at mass eateries that emerged in Japanese cities in the early twentieth century.[54] Moreover, from the 1930s onwards, Korean beef contributed to the build-up of Japanese armed forces in Manchuria. Japanese policymakers calculated that a fivefold increase in the export of Korean cattle to Manchuria (against 2,000 in 1937) would be needed to facilitate Japanese expansion into China.[55]

Unlike in the case of the provisioning of the Japanese armed forces with Korean beef at the time of the Russo-Japanese War three decades earlier, Korean cattle were now processed in Korea itself rather than first being transported to Japan. Statistical data on beef production and processing on the Korean peninsula for the second half of the 1930s reveals that the number of cows slaughtered for meat in Korea nearly doubled between 1938 and 1939, from 4,472,435 to 8,331,305 head.[56] This drastic increase corresponds with dramatic growth in the production of canned beef, from less than 0.5 million kg in 1938 to over 1 million kg the following year.[57] A closer look into the geographical distribution of the slaughterhouses and canned beef manufacturers reveals that they operated in close proximity to each other; the processing centres of Korean beef were located in the North Kyŏngsang and South Chŏlla provinces in the southern part of the peninsula. The third largest concentration of slaughterhouses and the well-developed canning industry were in South Hamgyŏng Province in the north. We may surmise that the more than 2 million head of cattle slaughtered there in the peak year of 1939, and the over 1.5 million in both 1938 and 1940, were shipped from the port of Hŭngnam, one of the largest in the colony.

The rapidly rising volume of exported Korean beef corresponds with the build-up of the Imperial Japanese Army on the Asian continent. The troop strength of Kwantung Army in Manchuria increased from two to four divisions between 1931 and 1935, and swelled to thirteen divisions (with a total manpower of 700,000 combat troops) at the peak of its strength in 1941.[58] Beef was not the only source of protein that Korea supplied to the soldiers of the Imperial Japanese Army. The Japanese troops stationed in Manchuria and China contracted a growing share of the production of the Korean seafood canneries. In terms of volume it was Korean pilchards and sardines, rather than Korean beef, that sustained Japanese soldiers stationed overseas. The outbreak of the Second Sino-Japanese War in 1937 corresponded with a dramatic increase in the volume of production of seafood canning in the colony, from 8,949,025 kg in 1937 to 13,027,014 kg in 1939.[59] The same holds true for the volume of exports, which nearly tripled in 1937 in relation to the previous year, and nearly tripled again between 1937 and 1939 (from 357,193 to 998,107 dozen cans).[60]

Seafood canning was the largest and most profitable branch of the Korean canning industry throughout the colonial period, and in the 1930s canned sardines (pilchards) took the lead as its most important product. Four different varieties were manufactured: sardines in tomato sauce, sardines flavoured with soy sauce and ginger, sardines *au naturel* and sardines flavoured with chilli powder. At first sardines in tomato sauce were clearly the bestseller; in 1936 this product comprised 96 per cent of all canned sardine sales.[61] During the following years, the production of sardines flavoured with chilli increased: in 1940, production was 3.6 times the size it had been in 1939. This dramatic increase might imply that consumption of canned sardines grew among Koreans as the food shortage unfolded (see chapter Four).

The importance of sardines for the Korean fisheries can be best understood in comparison with the total volume of catches. In 1935 sardines constituted 89 per cent of all seafood caught in Korea, followed by mackerel (9.4 per cent) and crab (0.7 per cent); topshell, abalone, whale and eel together made up the remaining 1 per cent. During 1937 and 1939, the most productive years for Korean fisheries, the share of sardines rose to 94 per cent, while mackerel dropped to less than 5 per cent and the catch of crab declined by half.[62]

It must be pointed out that canning was only a marginal method of utilizing the phenomenal catch of Korean sardines, which served as the chief resource for the fish oil and fish meal industry established by Japanese entrepreneurs in the early 1920s. Production tripled between 1935 and 1940, reaching the value of 115,000,000 yen that year.[63] More than 2,000 small sardine-oil fertilizer factories, run mainly by Koreans, operated on the Korean east coast. The colony supplied Japan with three-quarters of its fish oil, which in wartime had a wide range of strategic applications, from acting as a substitute fuel to being a major ingredient in the production of glycerine and gunpowder.

Before the spectacular growth of the catching and processing of sardines, canned crab ranked as the most profitable item of the Korean canning industry. Canned crabmeat was the true success story of the Japanese canning industry. From the late 1920s onwards it dominated the American market.[64] The bulk of crab for export was caught in the waters of Hokkaido, Kamchatka and Southern Sakhalin, and processed immediately on specialized canning ships. The crab canneries in Korea were clustered on the northeastern shore of the peninsula in South Hamgyŏng Province and Kangwŏn Province.[65] They were set up and operated by the Japanese entrepreneurs who had previously been active in Hokkaido and Sakhalin.

Within only two years, between 1938 and 1940, the production of canned crab dropped by nearly 60 per cent and never recovered.[66] The share of crab in the total value of canned seafood exported by Korea diminished accordingly. In 1936 it still accounted for over 36

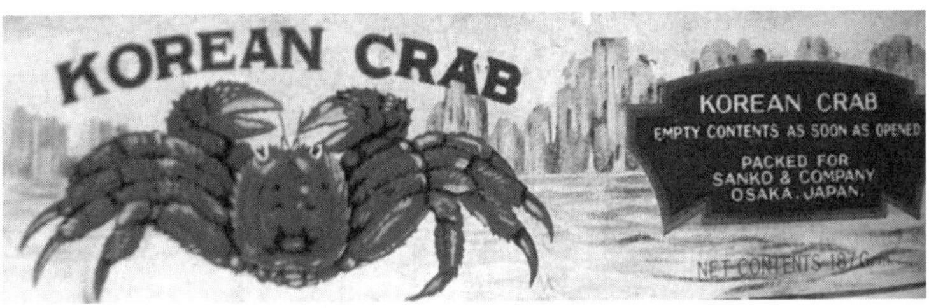

Korean crabs canned for export, 1931.

per cent of the total export value, and in 1937, 41 per cent. However, two years later the share dropped to a mere 11 per cent.[67] In a world of total war and food shortages there was no longer a role for upmarket commodities like crab.

2

Consumption Colonized

Living in the Colonial City

Unlike colonial powers that relied heavily on native administrators, the Japanese colonial governments and Japanese corporations imported large amounts of human capital from Japan – competent and loyal personnel who were placed in high and lower ranks of the colonial establishment to manage the government and the economy. The geographical proximity of metropole and colony greatly encouraged this trend. By 1939 the Japanese population in Korea had reached 650,000 – around 3 per cent of the entire population of the colony (see p. 175, Table 1). This colonists-to-colonized ratio is remarkable when compared to 0.2 per cent in French Indochina, 0.7 per cent in British Malaya and 0.4 per cent in the Netherlands East Indies.[1]

Japanese migrants first began to settle in the newly established treaty ports soon after the 'opening' of Korea in 1876. Unlike the flow of migrants pre-1910, who were mainly poor adventurers seeking rapid enrichment, urban middle-class professionals formed the majority of the Japanese population during the colonial period. The engineers, accountants, bureaucrats and entrepreneurs who arrived on Korean soil in growing numbers after 1910 belonged to the class that ardently embraced the hybrid Japanese-Western mass culture that began to emerge in urban Japan after the turn of the twentieth century. They wore Western-style suits, shopped at department stores, frequented the cinema and enjoyed other forms of Western mass culture that had by the 1920s become integrated into the everyday practice of middle-class Japanese urbanites.[2]

Since Japanese settlers were nearly 70 per cent urban, while 90 per cent of Koreans lived in rural areas, the Japanese presence in large cities like Pusan, Pyongyang, Taegu and Inch'ŏn by far exceeded the average 3 per cent ratio: in the colonial capital of Keijō they exceeded 20 per

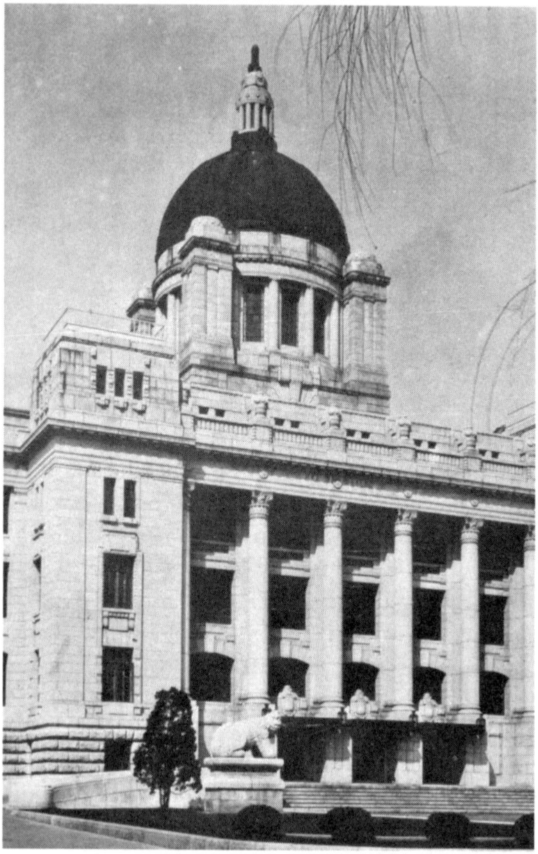

Government-General building in Keijō (Seoul), a symbol of Japanese colonial rule, *c.* 1939.

cent.[3] Thus the needs, fashions and tastes of Japanese expatriates shaped the urban landscape in colonial Korea to a considerable degree.

Needless to say, the new urban infrastructure developed by the Japanese significantly altered the experience of urban living for Koreans as well.[4] An important aim of the urban planners of the colonial capital was to astound Korean residents. Monumental architecture, largely inspired by European and American examples, served as a symbol of Japanese superiority. Major road projects completed during the first phase of urban reforms between 1913 and 1917 connected the southern part of the city, where Japanese settlers tended to reside, with a traditional core of the pre-colonial capital, north of the Ch'ŏnggyech'ŏn stream.[5] While the stream symbolically divided the colonial capital into a 'backward', predominantly Korean-inhabited northern

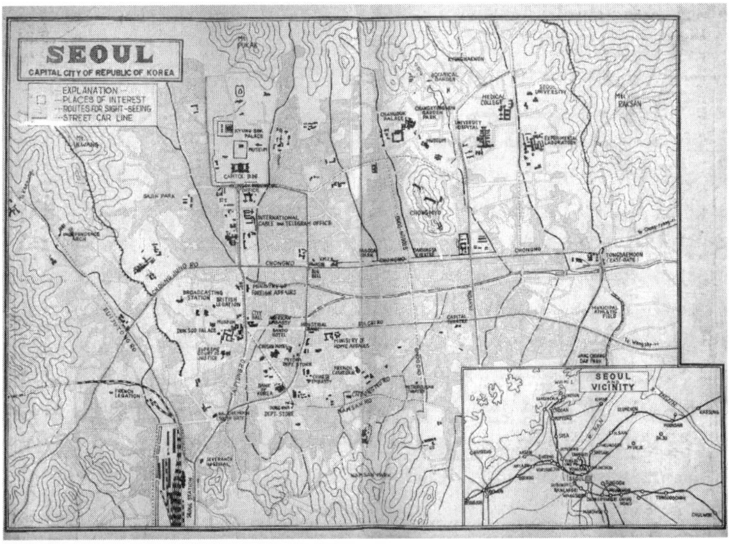

A map of central Seoul from the late 1940s or early 1950s, still reflecting the colonial structure of the capital, with governmental offices and department stores located in the southern half of the city. Taihei Avenue features under its Korean pronunciation, 'Taipyungro'.

half and a 'modern', Japanized southern half, the city's axis, the newly constructed Taihei Avenue, linked the two together, juxtaposing the contrast. During the second stage of urban reforms in 1919–24 the avenue was linked via the newly constructed Han River Bridge with the main traffic route to the port of Inch'ŏn to the south. Northwards, it continued towards the monumental Government-General building constructed in the heart of the Korean neighbourhoods on the grounds of the royal palace of the Chosŏn Dynasty (1392–1910). As Todd Henry argues in his study of colonial Seoul, Taihei Avenue came to reflect

> Japanese colonial power in its various manifestations: political (Government-General building on Kyŏngbok Palace grounds), economic (Honmachi and South Gate commercial district), transportational (Keijō train station), spiritual (Keijō and Chōsen shrines on Namsan), and military (Yongsan army headquarters).[6]

The newly emerging modern landscape of Keijō included not only wide roads, electric street cars and the monumental architecture of government buildings but new forms of public entertainment, such as cinemas, department stores, restaurants and cafés. Inevitably the hybrid Japanese-Western urban mass culture reproduced in the colony was perceived differently by the Japanese and Korean residents. Generally speaking, the latter enjoyed a much lower standard of living, and, apart from a handful of Koreans who had had an opportunity to travel abroad, they were entirely unfamiliar with the conveniences and trappings of the modern city before the colonial culture of consumption developed during the 1930s. With the exception of the domestic help employed in Japanese households, the colonized and the colonizers led separate lives, rarely interacting with each other.[7] However, the growing public space of the colonial city increasingly provided a setting for encounters, if not interaction: a world in which the boundaries of the colonial framework could be temporarily transcended.

Dining out in Keijō

According to the records of Keijō's Chamber of Commerce in 1939, over 250 establishments serving food and drink operated in the capital at the time.[8] The records divided these establishments into several categories, the largest being Japanese-style restaurants (73), followed by cafés (55), so-called *shokudō* or cafeterias (34), bars (30), Japanese restaurants specializing in a specific dish such as *sukiyaki*, sushi or *udon* noodles (23), Korean-style eateries and pubs (22), tea rooms (9), Korean-style restaurants (8), Western-style restaurants (5) and Chinese-style restaurants (4). The list compiled by the Chamber of Commerce was far from complete, which is evident when one considers the much larger membership of restaurant guilds active in the capital at exactly the same time. For example: the Restaurant Business Association of Keijō (Keijō Ryōriya Eigyō Kumiai) counted 44 members, the Association of Keijō Cafeterias (Keijō Shokudō Kumiai) 250 members, the Japanese and Western Food Association of Chongno (Keijō Shōro Wayōshoku Kumiai) 70 members, the Western Food Business Association of Keijō (Keijō Seiyō Ryōrigyō Kumiai) 80 members, the Japanese and Western Food Business Association of Eastern Keijō (Keijō Tōbu Wayō Ryōrigyō Kumiai) 41 members, the Chongno Association of Korean-owned Restaurants (Keijō Shōro Chōjin Inshokuten Kumiai) 270 members, the Restaurant Association of Western Keijō (Keijō Seibu Inshokuten Kumiai) 107 members, and the Restaurant Association of Southern Keijō (Keijō Seibu Inshokuten Kumiai) 140 members.[9] Moreover, the figures included neither the food peddlers who sold a variety of snacks throughout the city nor the restaurants and eating houses run by Chinese immigrants.[10]

These inaccuracies notwithstanding, the Chamber of Commerce's records compellingly demonstrate both that by the late 1930s Keijō offered its citizens a wide range of options for dining out, and that the city's gastronomic scene had acquired a highly multicultural character. This development was closely related to the Japanese penetration of the country since the late nineteenth century. A steady flow of Japanese migrants, and later colonists, resulted in the spread of facilities and services that were considered essential for maintaining a Japanese lifestyle, including those related to food.[11] Restaurants, inns and brothels were among the first enterprises that sprang up in the Japanese residential areas to cater to the needs of their (at the time overwhelmingly male) clientele. As early as 1888, Seoul counted five Japanese liquor shops, ten Japanese-style confectioners and fourteen Japanese restaurants.[12]

The arrival of Japanese restaurants indirectly stimulated the growth of Korean native gastronomy – the *yoritchip* ('eating house' or restaurant) and the *siktang* ('cafeteria') are modern, twentieth-century constructs. A highly differentiated restaurant culture comparable to that of Paris or Edo (present-day Tokyo) had not developed in pre-modern Korea. Taverns and food stalls that operated at markets, commonly known as *chumak* or *kaekchujip*, were the chief gastronomic establishments, serving simple food to hungry travellers and providing a site where male customers could have a drink with a few snacks.[13] Posh bordellos, in which upper-class (*yangban*) men were entertained by refined courtesans (*kisaeng*), also served drinks with snacks, but began to develop into restaurants only after the turn of the twentieth century. One of the most famous establishments of this sort was Myŏngwŏlgwan, founded in 1909 by An Sun-Hwan, a former chef at the Korean royal palace. 'His formula for success', as Andrei Lankov explains,

> was based on a combination of the sophisticated palace cuisine (quite different from ordinary Korean cuisine) and the best available girls. Indeed guests were treated to the same food that was once enjoyed by kings while being entertained by the most beautiful kisaengs in the Korean capital. An also employed a former royal liquor-maker

> whose liquors were legendary . . . The first houses of haute cuisine were extremely exclusive and well beyond the means of the average Korean. For example, a simple dinner in *Myŏngwŏlgwan* cost the equivalent of an average monthly salary![14]

Around the time when such exclusive Korean restaurants began to emerge, at the other end of the gastronomic spectrum, cheap Chinese eateries run by Chinese immigrants slowly started to gain popularity among Korean customers. Statistical records reveal that in 1922 over 600 Chinese restaurants were operating in eleven major cities throughout Korea.[15] Since most immigrants hailed from Shandong Province, the Korean version of Chinese cuisine that began to develop in colonial Korea was based on the traditions of northeast China. *Chajangmyŏn*, a noodle dish that by the late twentieth century had grown into a symbol of Chinese cuisine in South Korea, is reported to have originated in a 'Chinese restaurant, Gonghwachun, which opened in Incheon in 1905'.[16] The influence of Japanese restaurateurs who set up Chinese restaurants in the colony has also had a lasting impact on Chinese-style dining in Korea: for example, pickled giant white radish or mooli (*takuanzuke*) – one of the most ubiquitous Japanese pickles – still appears on the side of every dish served in Chinese restaurants in South Korea today. Moreover, several names of dishes on their menus, such as *udong*, *tchamppong* and *yakki mandu*, are of Japanese origin.[17]

Japanese influences were particularly pronounced in Western-style colonial restaurants. By the 1920s Japanese residents in Korean cities had managed to fully recreate the gastronomic scene of the homeland, which had by then become highly eclectic. A characteristic feature of twentieth-century Japanese urban gastronomy was its three-tiered Japanese/Western/Chinese structure. This structure implied that along with traditional Japanese establishments, Western-style and Chinese-style restaurants were ubiquitous and available at various price ranges. Modern, large-scale eateries such as the ones operating at train terminals and at department stores customarily served all three cuisines.[18]

Along with Korean, Japanese, and Chinese food, Western-style cuisine also became available in the colony. Generally speaking, the spread of Western gastronomy in Korea was only marginally related to direct influences from Europe and the United States. Like other aspects of Korean modernity, the construction of Western food in Korea was mediated by a Japanese filter. The use of the term *yangsik* ('Western food') is largely influenced by the Japanese category of *yōshoku*, with its twofold meaning: on the one hand, it is a neutral term referring to European and American cuisines generally, with a strong emphasis on the Anglo-Saxon culinary tradition due to the overwhelming British and American presence in East Asia since the late nineteenth century. On the other hand, the term came to signify domesticated versions of selected British and American dishes featured on the menus of the cheap Western-style restaurants that became ubiquitous in Japanese cities after the turn of the twentieth century.[19] Recipes for these Japanese–Western hybrids soon appeared in Korean cookbooks, clearly influenced by the Japanese publications. A Western Food appendix in one of the first modern Korean cookbooks, *Chosŏn yori chebŏp* ('Korean Recipes'), published in 1924, included recipes for fried rice (*furaido raisu*), chicken rice (*chikin raisu*) and curry on rice (*karē raisu*).[20] Along with the names of the dishes, ingredients of Western origin are often referred to in this book by their Japanese names rather than the Western originals: onion and curry powder, for example.

It must be pointed out that the very first Western-style restaurants that emerged in Korea during the early years of the twentieth century were an exception to the 'Japanese filter' rule. The pioneering establishment was Sontag Hotel, run by a Russian woman of German origin, Antoinette Sontag (1854–1925), who had arrived in Korea in the 1880s, accompanying her sister, who was married to Karl Weber (1841–?), the first Russian envoy to Seoul.[21] In 1902 she secured permission from King Kojong (1852–1919) to establish a hotel to accommodate foreign guests of the Imperial Korean Household. For this purpose the court gave her a three-storey brick building which had initially served as a Western-style reception hall for foreign diplomats.

Sontag Hotel was modelled on similar establishments throughout Asia that provided lodging for genteel travellers from Europe and the United States. Following the established conventions of the time, the hotel operated a restaurant which served French-style meals.[22] In 1909, when Sontag left Korea and the hotel was taken over by a Frenchman, J. Boher (already the proprietor of two other Western-style hotels in Seoul, Central Hotel and Palace Hotel), Sontag Hotel was advertised in *The Seoul Press* as 'the largest and most convenient hotel in Korea', offering 'every home comfort for family and tourist visitors and finest French cuisine'.[23] Since Lankov reports that Sontag served homemade Russian meals rather than French cuisine in her hotel, and that some of her guests perceived the establishment as lacking in sophistication, it is plausible that it is Boher who should be credited for the culinary erudition of Sontag Hotel, not Sontag herself.[24]

By 1914, in concert with the colonial encroachment on the peninsula, the Japanese-owned Chōsen Hotel stripped Sontag Hotel of its reputation as Keijō's best hotel, in culinary terms as in other amenities. This grand hotel, newly erected in 1914, became a showcase of the Japanese 'civilizing mission', the epitome of Western-style convenience and sophistication in the Far East. Along with such modern conveniences as steam-heated bedrooms with attached bathrooms, electric lights and fans, the hotel offered outstanding dining facilities.[25] *Terry's Guide to the Japanese Empire*, published in 1933, describes it as

> Best in the city. Recommended. Modern, fire- and earthquake proof. Member of the Japan Hotel Association. Many comforts and modern conveniences. Telephones, radio, moving pictures, good food, and service. English spoken.[26]

The regular dining room had the capacity to serve breakfast, lunch and dinner simultaneously to up to 90 customers, and the hotel also operated a private dining room for smaller parties and a large banqueting- and ballroom that could accommodate up to 300 guests. In the winter months (between November and February) the banqueting room was usually fully booked for wedding parties, and during the rest of the year it frequently hosted official banquets organized for the leading

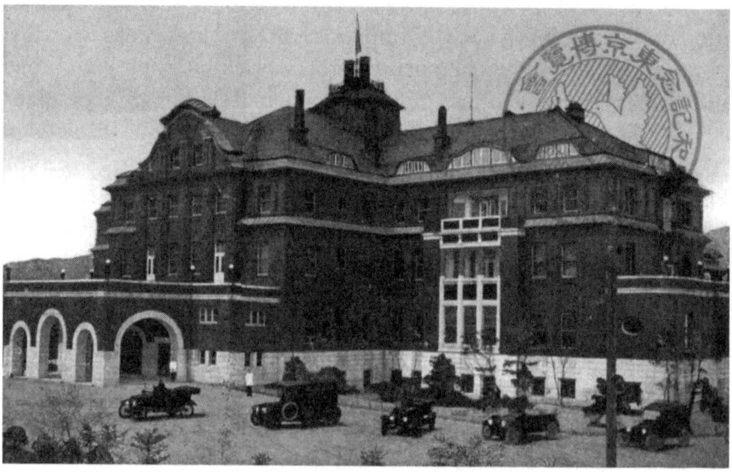

The Chōsen Hotel in Keijō, 1922.

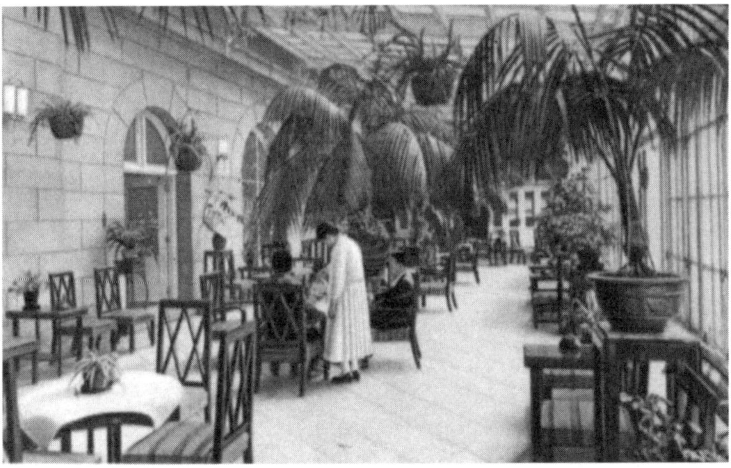

The Sun Lounge at the Chōsen Hotel, Keijō, 1930s.

members of the colonial establishment, such as the office of the Governor-General or the Keijō Chamber of Commerce.[27]

Since the Chōsen Hotel was a clear marker of distinction, the Japanese and Korean elites were regular guests of the hotel's restaurant. The regular dining room is reported to have been a favourite spot for posh ladies to gather for afternoon tea, sandwiches, confectionery and ice cream.[28] The exclusive character of the Chōsen Hotel dining room was reflected in its prices. In around 1933 it charged 1.75 yen for breakfast, 2.5 yen for tiffin and 3 yen for dinner, while the restaurant inside the Keijō Railway Station served Western-style lunch and dinner for half that price. Cafeteria Aokidō was famous for its economical 0.5 yen lunch, while a budget eatery inside the Keijō City Hall charged a mere 0.2–0.35 yen for a Western-style, and 0.22 yen for a Japanese-style, meal.[29]

Tourist guidebooks are an invaluable source of information on the gastronomic scene of colonial Seoul. The Japan Tourist Bureau (JTB), established at the Japanese Imperial Railways Corporate Head Office in 1912, opened colonial outposts in Taiwan, Manchuria and Korea the same year. It played a coordinating role in promoting Korea as a tourist destination, including the organization from 1918 onwards of innovative packaged tours with discounted steamship passage tickets, railway passes and hotel coupons. The guidebooks for the colonies published by the Japan Tourist Bureau, the Government-General of Korea office and South Manchurian Railways were all

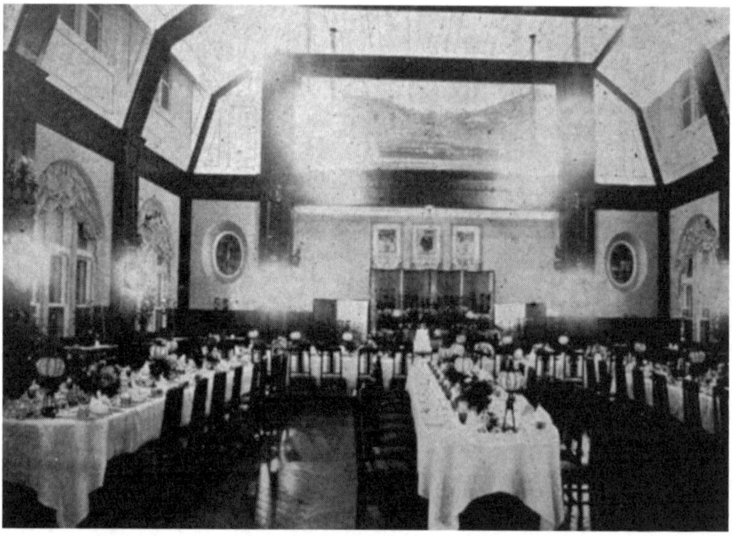

The ballroom and banqueting hall of the Chōsen Hotel, Keijō, *c.* 1930s.

modelled after Victorian-era handbooks on Japan, and included practical information, such as transportation fees, admissions to museums and the costs of food at recommended restaurants, alongside descriptions of scenic, cultural and business destinations.[30] A tourist guidebook to Keijō of 1936 recommended several Western-style restaurants, including top-end establishments such as the Chōsen Hotel and Honmachi Hotel, Chiyoda Grill and Ch'ŏngmoktang (Aokidō). The last is allegedly the oldest, and at the time was the most exclusive Western-style restaurant in Keijō. It opened in 1909 as a branch of a Tokyo business. Along with the restaurant, it operated an exclusive grocery store, housed in a handsome four-storey building in the centre of the business district at Nandaimon Avenue.[31]

The Japanese guidebook to the colonial capital of 1936 also recommended cheaper cafeterias, such as Kagetsu, Nikoniko and the cafeteria at the Keijō Railway Station, where broader segments of the tourist population could afford to dine.[32] Kagetsu managed a chain of different kinds of dining establishments bearing this name: the original Kagetsu, also referred to as the 'main store' (*honten*), an upmarket Japanese-style restaurant situated at the very centre of the Honmachi entertainment district; the elegant Kagetsu Villa, located in the serene surroundings of Nanzan Park at the southern edge of the city; and the convenient Kagetsu cafeteria, which operated on the second floor of

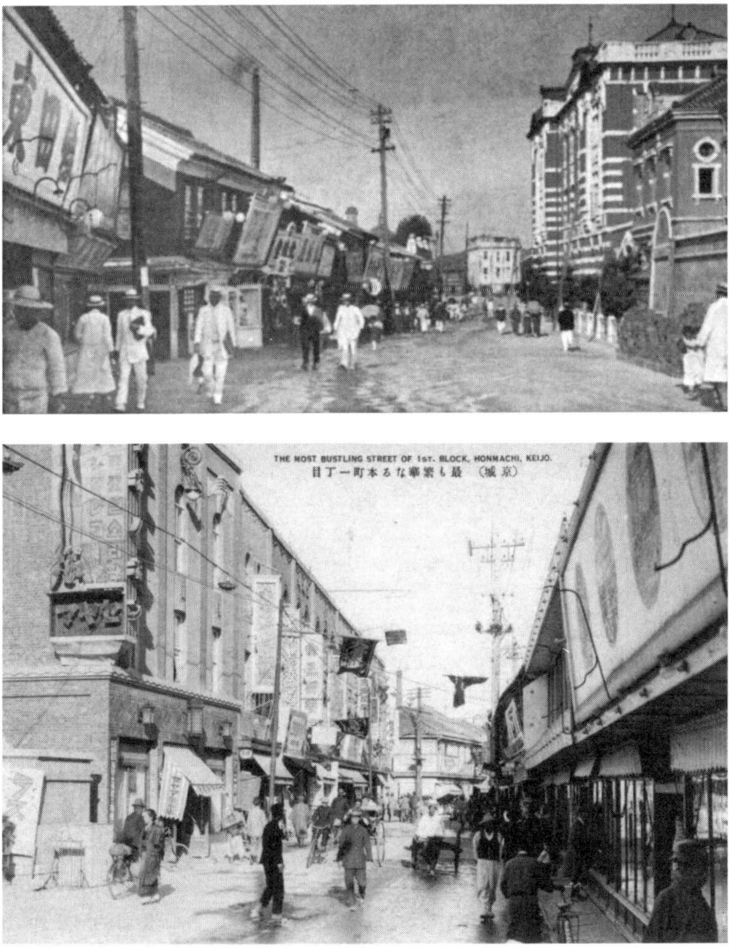
THE MOST BUSTLING STREET OF 1st. BLOCK, HONMACHI, KEIJO.
最も繁華なる本町一丁目 (京城)

Honmachi, the most fashionable shopping district in Keijō, *c.* 1930s.

the Nissei Building in Koganemachi district and had a capacity of 70–80 diners.[33] All three are listed in a tourist booklet about Keijō published by the Keijō Tourism Association in 1934 among the restaurants, cafeterias, cafés and tea rooms recommended for Japanese tourists (see p. 175, Table 11).

By the 1930s, as well as Japanese residents and tourists, dining establishments that served Korean, Japanese, Chinese and Western food became part of the daily life of Korean urbanites, as a diary of a Korean intellectual, Mun Il-p'yŏ, testified in 1934.[34] Between January and

December of that year Mun Il-p'yŏ recorded in his diary a visit to a restaurant or a pub on 101 days, which would translate into eating or drinking out every 3–4 days, sometimes visiting more than one establishment on a single day. Mun patronized all four types of food available in colonial Seoul, with Korean eateries and pubs featuring most frequently (49 entries), followed by Western-style (29), Chinese (24) and Japanese (13) establishments. Along with restaurants and pubs that are recorded only once or twice, Mun seems to have his favourites to which he often returns, such as the Chinese eateries (Ch'ŏng yoritchip, Taegwanwŏn and Wŏnhŭngru), and the Korean-style Taeryŏngwan and Uch'ungwan. Interestingly, the restaurant mentioned most often in the diary is San'in shokudō (Sangwŏn siktang), which served hybrid Japanese-Western food. It appears for the first time in the entry of 2 August and then follows 25 times, often almost on a daily basis (2 and 3 August, 11, 12 and 14 October, 2, 3, 6, 13, 16, 19, 20 and 23 November, 14 and 16 December). Mun dined in the upmarket Western-style restaurant of the Chōsen Hotel only once (on 2 February), and at the celebrated Myŏngwŏlgwan at three occasions (5 May and 9 and 11 December).[35]

The ubiquitous presence of cafés, bars, eateries and department store restaurants is also widely reflected in colonial-period Korean fiction. The narrative of the novel *Three Generations* includes dialogues staged in Japanese noodle shops, Western-style restaurants and hybrid Western-Japanese bars and cafés.[36] The cafeteria at the Keijō Rail Station features in Yi Sang's celebrated novel *Wings*, and unemployed intellectual P – the protagonist of Ch'ae Man-Shik's novel *A Ready-made Life* – 'depending on the amount of money in hand . . . might have Chinese pancakes, beef-and-rice soup, or even a Western-style lunch in a department store'.[37] The conspicuous appearance of such establishments, along with other kinds of modern urban infrastructure, as a context for modernist Korean fiction highlights their very novelty.[38] Nonetheless, their presence throughout the city and – more importantly – their popularity among their Korean clientele reveals the transformative impact of (Japanese) consumer culture on (Korean) colonial society.

Restaurants located in department stores were definitely the trendiest spots for dining out in 1930s Keijō. Several factors were responsible for their popularity. First, they were particularly prized for the value-for-money of their menus.[39] Moreover, they offered a choice between Japanese, Chinese and Western dishes. The Korean-owned

Hwasin department store also served Korean-style meals along with Japanese- and Western-style dishes.[40] The appeal of multicultural menus notwithstanding, it seems unlikely that the food was the sole or even the most important reason behind the tremendous popularity of department store restaurants.

Department stores in Keijō usually outsourced the cooking itself to professional restaurateurs who dispatched their cooking staff to the department stores' kitchens. At the Mitsukoshi department store only Western-style dishes and drinks were prepared by its own staff. The restaurant Kikuya (from Nanzanmachi) took charge of Japanese-style dishes and noodles; Kawachō restaurant (from Asahimachi) was responsible for Chinese cuisine, tempura and eel specialities; and sushi came from the renowned Sushikyū in Meijimachi. In the case of Minakai department store, preparation of Japanese and Western dishes was outsourced to Kagetsu restaurant, and Chinese food and noodles to the restaurant Benke.[41] The prices of meals oscillated around 1 yen depending on the item, which was comparable to other establishments that operated throughout the city.

It seems plausible that the splendid interiors, superb service and modern ambience of the department store restaurants constituted their chief added value. They were much grander than comparable eateries elsewhere in Keijō. For example, the restaurant of the Mitsukoshi department store was able simultaneously to serve 130–150 customers, and its competitors – the Chōjiya and Minakai department stores – up to 180–200 customers.[42] An additional attraction was the fact that these restaurants were usually situated on the top floors of multi-storey modern buildings. The restaurant of the Minakai store, for example, newly constructed in 1933, was famous for its magnificent view. It was located on the sixth floor, which was the highest dining site in the entire city. Customers were transported to these unusual locations by elevators – in itself a fascinating experience for most diners. Waitresses dressed in Western-style uniforms – all eighteen years old or younger – completed the bewildering picture.

The turnout at department store restaurants in Keijō was relatively high. On average, approximately 1,000 customers dined at each restaurant on weekdays, and the number often doubled on Sundays and holidays.[43] For comparison, Selfridges, a leading department store in early twentieth-century London, operated a restaurant that served between 2,000 and 3,000 patrons a day.[44] In the United States, Marshall Field's department store in Chicago had a large tearoom, 'seating five hundred

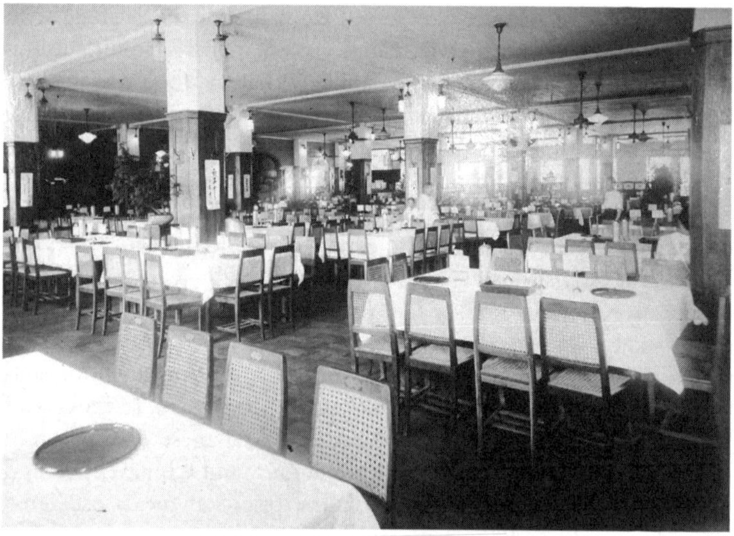

The interior of a department store cafeteria, *c.* 1930s.

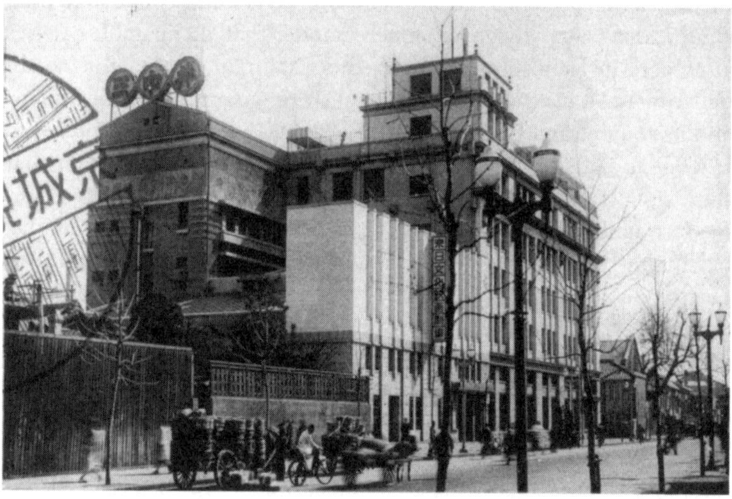

Exterior view of the Minakai department store in Keijō, *c.* 1930s.

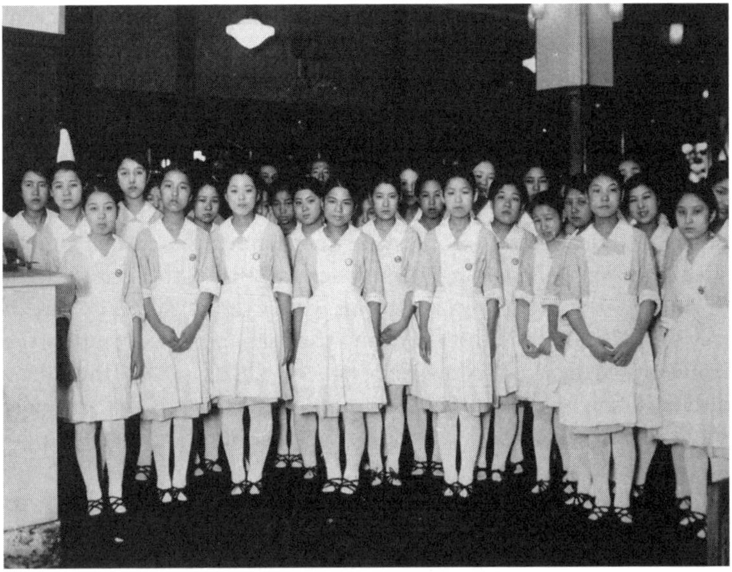

Young waitresses dressed in Western-style uniform were a characteristic feature of department store cafeterias in Japan and Korea in the first decades of the 20th century.

for afternoon tea, from three to five in the afternoon on the fourth floor'.[45] As was the case in Europe, the United States and Japan, the popularity of department store restaurants in colonial Korea seems to have only partly been related to the gustatory pleasure. Since comparable food was served in other restaurants throughout the city, it seems that what appealed most to the Japanese and Korean crowds who frequented department store dining halls was an opportunity to enter the 'dream world' of commodities. Labelled 'palaces of consumption' and 'lands of desire' by contemporary observers, department stores used their restaurants to lure customers onto their premises.

The Department Store as a Vanguard of Mass Consumption

There seems to be a general consensus among scholars concerning the role of the department store – originating in Paris and soon recreated in other European countries, North America and Western colonial enclaves – as the vanguard of consumer culture.[46] The department store provoked desires and feelings towards things, becoming a place where customers went to be entertained by commodities, where selling was mingled with amusement. The chief validation behind its phenomenal influence was the simple fact that it allowed consumers to 'indulge temporarily in the fantasy of wealth'.[47]

As it did elsewhere in Asia,[48] the department store in Korea served as a central stage for the development of a modern culture of consumption in the colonial cities. It was the quintessential modern urban space where new practices and attitudes were being born. Focusing on the dining facilities operated by the department stores, this chapter aims to shed light on a phenomenon that one might label the 'colonization of consumption'. The power relations within the consumer culture of colonial Korea during the 1930s and the early '40s vividly reflect the ambiguity of the lived colonial experience. While Koreans (the colonized) willingly embraced the colonizer as a trendsetter, the economic survival of the Japanese department stores was often dependent on the patronage of the Korean public.

Lower prices and the large selection of commodities displayed under one roof only partly explain the success of the new stores that began to thrive in Europe and North America towards the end of the nineteenth century. Much more significant was the fact that each item on sale was marked with a fixed price and that customers were encouraged to inspect the merchandise even if they did not (intend to) make a purchase. This was a revolutionary idea indeed, since prices in retail shops had thus far been subject to negotiation and it was difficult for a buyer to back out once the negotiations began. In other words, the department store introduced an entirely new dimension to shopping by providing the customer with the freedom to browse, 'the liberty to indulge in dreams without being obliged to buy'.[49] But the new consumer culture nurtured inside department stores entailed much more than changing practices related to purchasing commodities. The marketing strategies of the large-scale nineteenth-century retailers – aimed in the first place at elevating profit – cultivated an entirely new consciousness among their customers by inflaming a continuing desire for the new, and creating a novel public space in which shopping functioned as a form of entertainment.[50] A defining principle in designing these spaces was the emphasis on its distance from the ordinary. By utilizing cutting-edge technology and modernist architecture, department stores became surreal visions of utopian modern life. Alternatively, through the use of exotic decor they could temporarily be transformed into one or another Oriental fantasy world. In the U.S., Leach explains, 'depending on the fashion of the month or year, each particular subtheme might be Islamic, Indian, Japanese, or Chinese, with stores decorated as mosques, temples or desert oases'.[51] Along with stressing distance from the ordinary, Turkish rugs, Oriental silks and Venetian lanterns conveyed a sense of lavishness and had a highly seductive effect which in turn underscored the department store's imagery as a 'dream world' or a 'land of desire'.[52]

As department stores began to be transplanted into Asia in the early twentieth century, the imagery of the department store as a surreal fantasy world became even more pronounced without any need for such Orientalizing strategies. The multi-storeyed, grand, unfamiliar-looking buildings themselves, with their escalators, lifts and revolving doors, epitomized exoticism and were far removed from the everyday reality of the Asian populations.[53] In Japan, along with introducing the population to the world of fashion, brands and good taste, department stores performed the additional role of an educator: they informed the public about Western architecture, technology and culture. Furthermore, as Louise Young explains, they 'promoted themselves as sites for novel urban entertainment and created recreational spaces that celebrated a notion of leisure built around consumption'.[54] In their quest to create the new concept of recreational space, Japanese department stores devoted large amounts of floor space and lavish resources to creating lounges, restaurants, exhibition galleries, roof gardens, roller-skating rinks, children's playgrounds and even miniature zoos. 'Such spaces', Young argues, 'enunciated an idea of leisure that incorporated recreation into a daily ritual of consumption.'[55] As symbols of the West and triumphant visions of the modern, Japanese department stores also functioned as tourist attractions – becoming themselves 'sites of consumption' in every sense of the word.[56]

These characteristics of Japanese department stores were recreated, down to minute details, in colonial Korea. The first retailer to proclaim itself a '*paekhwajŏm*' was Mitsukoshi – already a pioneer of the department store business in Japan.[57] It opened a sales office (*shutchōjo*) in Keijō in 1916, which twelve years later was transformed into a branch (*shiten*). In October 1930 Mitsukoshi moved into a splendid, newly constructed building opposite the Keijō Post Office, the current Shinsegye department store.[58] Sales at the new Keijō *shiten* were comparable to those of the branch in Osaka, the second largest city in Japan.[59]

Mitsukoshi was the only Japan-based department store that operated in Korea, and the Keijō branch was its only store in the colony. Other Japanese department stores in Korea were all local

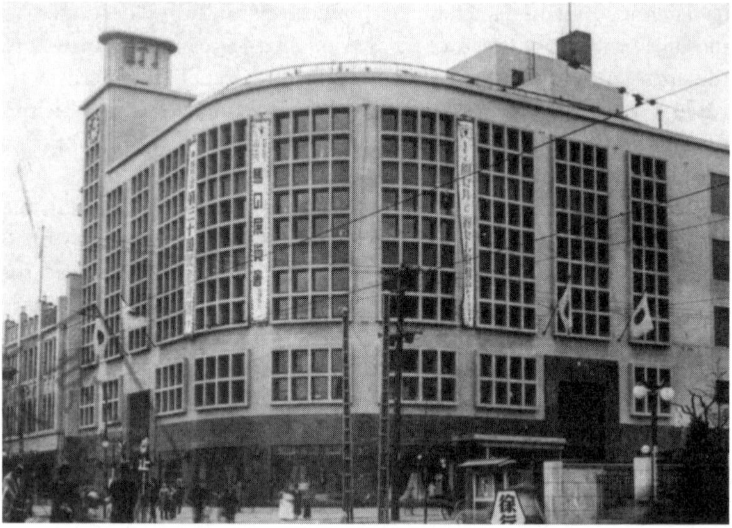

Exterior of the Chōjiya department store in Keijō, *c.* 1930s.

enterprises that managed a network of branch stores in major Korean cities, and later also expanded to Manchuria and China. Like the pioneering department stores in Europe and Japan, they originated from dry-goods enterprises. Chōjiya, which since 1904 had been a chief supplier of uniforms for the Japanese and Korean government and the Korean railway, was the first to follow in the footsteps of Mitsukoshi and proclaim itself a department store. This happened in 1921. Five years later, the Hirata department store opened its door to the public. It was a low-profile store that capitalized mainly on the bulk sale of low-priced commodities and did not invest in the monumental interior and amenities which became so representative of the department store experience in colonial Korea as elsewhere.[60] In 1929 Minakai joined the business and was soon to become the largest chain of department stores in the colony. It operated fully fledged stores in Pyongyang, Taegu (both opened in 1933) and Pusan (since 1937) and smaller branch stores in Poju, Kwangju, Mokp'o, Kunsan, Taejŏn, Wŏnsan, Hamhŭng and Hŭngnam.

Keijō in the 1930s was the heyday of department store culture in colonial Korea. One by one the stores moved to newly constructed, magnificent, multi-storey buildings – Chōjiya in 1929, Mitsukoshi in 1930 and Minakai in 1933. The last retailer that proclaimed itself a department store in the capital was the Tonga department store, which opened in 1932 and was later renamed Hwasin. Hwasin was the proud creation of Korean entrepreneur Pak Hŭng-sik and an amalgamation of the two Korean retail enterprises – Hwasin Sanghoe and Tonga Puin Sanghoe – that emerged in the 1920s in reaction to the encroachment of Japanese merchants in the colony.[61] In January 1935 the store vanished in the flames of an accidental fire, but it reopened in an even grander seven-storey form two and a half years later. The total floor space of the new Hwasin made it the largest in Korea, outshining even the Mitsukoshi store.[62]

The phenomenal growth in the popularity of department stores in 1930s Keijō can be best illustrated by the stores' tax records.[63] Between 1931 and 1942 the total amount of sales tax paid by all the department stores (including the discount store Hirata) increased more than five-fold – from 9,465 to 56,319 yen. Under the economic boom generated by the Sino-Japanese War, sales skyrocketed, doubling their revenues during the period 1939–42. The important role that department stores played in the construction of the consumer culture of colonial Korea is customarily downplayed as a chiefly 'Japanese for Japanese' phenomenon, implying that the Japanese retailing business was patronized mainly by Japanese customers. In reality the situation seems to have been the reverse. Based on the stores' records, business historian Hayashi Hiroshige argues that the Japanese department store businesses in Keijō (and elsewhere in colonial Korea for that matter), which were all replicating the Japanese model, were for 60–70 per cent dependent on their Korean clientele.[64] In his view, patronage by the Japanese population alone would not have sustained three fully fledged Japanese department stores. A similar conclusion had been reached by a 1930s contemporary who described the ongoing 'department store war' in Keijō for the journal *Chōsen oyobi Manshū* ('Korea and Manchuria'). Based on comparison with the U.S., which ranked in the early twentieth century as the country with the highest concentration of department stores in the world, he calculated that the Japanese department stores of Keijō could never survive without Korean consumers.[65]

Why did Korean customers patronize department stores? In November 1934 the Korean newspaper *Chosŏn Ilbo* ('Korean Daily News') evaluated a department store shopping experience based on an opinion poll conducted among its readers. Respondents cited the abundance and variety of goods on sale, as well as the feeling of security and trust, as the chief advantages of department store shopping, along with the convenience of home delivery and agreeable service.[66]

Various attempts by Korean retailers to win back their customers from the Japanese merchant houses confirms that even in the 1920s strict segregation along ethnic lines was not the defining principle of the consumer culture of colonial Korea.[67] This does not necessarily mean that the ethnic factor was entirely irrelevant. Hwasin clearly capitalized on its Korean identity and cultivated the notion that shopping at the Korean department store was a patriotic deed. The store was strategically situated in Chongno, the pre-colonial heart of the capital, thus distancing itself from the 'Japanese' part of the city south of the Ch'ŏnggyech'ŏn stream, where the other three major department stores were clustered. However, Pak Hŭng-sik did not create a new market, but capitalized on the already existing one. Most of the products on sale at Hwasin were branded commodities manufactured in Japan, the majority of Hwasin's managerial staff were Japanese and the entire business formula was an exact copy of the Japanese model.[68] And despite Hwasin's explicitly Korean identity, many Korean customers still chose to patronize Mitsukoshi because of its greater variety of goods and better facilities.[69]

Women and the Culture of Consumption in Colonial Korea

In Europe, shopping had already been established as a pleasurable social activity among the upper classes before the rise of the department store.[70] An early nineteenth-century British contemporary observer noted that 'when persons of distinction are in town, the usual employment of the ladies is to go a-shopping. This they do without actually wanting to purchase anything.'[71] If not the inventor of the idea of shopping as entertainment, the department store was certainly responsible for democratizing this experience. The mass production of non-essential consumer goods and ready-to-wear clothing, paired with the development of cheap and reliable means of transportation, played a critical role in this retail revolution. However, this transformation would not have been possible without the chief actors on the scene of 'dream worlds' – women.

As elsewhere, a key secret behind the commercial success of the department store in colonial Korea was the fact that it created comfortable and exciting yet socially acceptable ways for Korean women to actively participate in modern urban life. Still, this innovation did not unfold without consequences. As elsewhere, the new culture of consumption introduced by the department store had a transformative, emancipating effect on women.[72] This impact did not escape the attention of the Korean media. An edition of the daily *Chosŏn Ilbo* in 1930 lamented the selfish behaviour of female students in the capital. Immediately after passing their first exams – the report explained – they rushed to Mitsukoshi or Chōjiya to buy make-up without even giving a thought to the hardships that their families in the provinces endured to pay their tuition fees.[73] A column in the same newspaper in 1933 criticized the young generation of Korean housewives who neglected *kimch'i* making and other household chores and instead dragged their husbands and children to department store restaurants, unnecessarily straining the family budget.[74]

Such criticism expressed in the Korean media during the 1930s echoes concerns voiced in London a few decades earlier. British public opinion feared that the participation of women in urban commercial culture encouraged sexual, moral and social disorder.[75] Interestingly, the idea of women taking refreshments on the premises of the department store assumed a central place in the censure. Operating a restaurant as part of a retail store was a new idea that first emerged in nineteenth-century Paris when the very concept of the department store took shape.[76] Whiteley's was the first store in London to serve food and drink in its small refreshment room, following the Paris example. This innovation, introduced in 1872, inspired a heated public debate over acceptable feminine spaces and behaviour outside the private home and family circle. When accused of encouraging sexual, moral and social decay by luring women outside the respectable boundaries of the home, the store's management argued the opposite: that the new facilities offered by the department store protected women from entering 'places of ill-repute such as [a] public house to have a drink or other refreshment'.[77]

During the following decades, the idea of the department store as an extension of the drawing room, a safe refuge in the modern city where genteel women could socialize with other genteel women, became increasingly pronounced. Luxurious interiors with elaborate dining facilities, lavatories, reading and writing rooms and other services encouraged customers to spend an entire day shopping within these 'large comfortable retail palaces'.[78] This model was replicated in Japan and its colonies. In the late 1930s Hwasin and other department stores in Keijō offered their customers a range of services that one could expect from a reputable department store abroad. In close proximity to the entrance one could find the information stand that handled enquiries about the location of the departments, as well as selling tickets for public transport and coupon tickets to be used at the in-house restaurant. Nearby was located a cloakroom where one could deposit luggage for the duration of one's visit to the store. Resting areas and lifts made travelling between departments less tiring. Other facilities included dressing rooms, restrooms, powder rooms, telephone booths, a beauty parlour, a photographic studio, a hothouse and a space where one could admire small birds.[79] Spaces for taking refreshments completed the picture. Unlike the establishments that served pre-modern Korea which were exclusively male oriented, department store restaurants were targeted specifically at women and 'happy families'.[80] Thus for many Korean women a visit to a department store entailed an opportunity to dine out, which in itself was a new and exciting experience.

The very first department store restaurant in the U.S. was installed at Macy's in New York in 1878. It was located on the second floor and the menu was limited to cold food prepared off the premises supplemented by hot tea, coffee and chocolate. 'A cheerless offering by modern standards, perhaps,' comments Ralph Hower in a monograph on Macy's history, 'but a boon to the tired shopper of the 1870s and '80s whom progress had not yet supplied with convenient and inexpensive restaurants.'[81] Along with providing weary shoppers with refreshments, department store restaurants in time acquired an additional function: to attract customers to enter the store. They were usually subsidized, providing the food, the service and the ambience for less than would be the case had they not been part of the marketing strategies of the grand stores. In the U.S. department stores competed for customers by installing ever more extravagant dining settings, not infrequently causing financial liabilities for the owners.[82]

While the furnishing of those restaurants was definitely more luxurious than the dining rooms of the majority of their customers, it was not strikingly different from what they were accustomed to at home. For Korean and Japanese women, however, the interior of the department store restaurant was a far stretch from their traditional domestic setting. Sitting on chairs at a table in a large space, even sharing a meal with a member of the opposite sex, were entirely new to Korean women, who usually dined at home using individual trays and sitting on cushions. Men always ate separately from women and not infrequently housewives would take their meals in the kitchen.[83] A phenomenal novelty applied to the food served at department store restaurants, too. With the exception of the dining room at Hwasin, which also served Korean cuisine, the menus of department store restaurants in Korea were overwhelmingly foreign. Soups, cutlets, omelettes, macaroni and fritters on the menus of European and American department stores did not differ much from the daily fare of the shoppers there, but pork cutlet, vegetable salad and curry on rice would have been entirely unfamiliar to the Korean customers of department store restaurants unless they belonged to the exclusive circle of the cosmopolitan elite.[84]

In sum, department store restaurants in colonial Korea were designed, as elsewhere, with a double purpose in mind: to retain customers longer on the premises and to lure them into the store in the first place. Korean women ardently embraced department store restaurants for the very same reasons their counterparts in Europe and the U.S. did. However, they had additional reasons for excitement similar to those experienced by Japanese women. First of all, the food on the menu included dishes that they hardly had an opportunity to sample elsewhere; foreign food remained the domain of restaurants and professional caterers throughout the colonial period, practically never being prepared at home. Furthermore, the sleek and modern appeal of the Western-style buildings of the Korean department stores, and the interior of their dining halls, stood in strong contrast with the familiar surroundings of the Korean home. These differences underlined the juxtaposition of the multiple temporalities of colonial Korea: a relatively traditional, Korean life at home and the dazzling speed of change in the hybrid Japanese-Western public life of the city.

Department Stores and Colonial Modernity in Korea

As elsewhere, the department store played a crucial role in the construction of a modern culture of consumption in Korea. It was ardently embraced by Korean urbanites despite its association with Japanese colonial oppression. By 1941, for example, the sales of the Keijō branch of the Mitsukoshi department store doubled that of the store in Sapporo, which was comparable in size.[85] In principle, Korean subjects of the Japanese Empire did not differ from shoppers elsewhere who had been bewitched by the seductive spells of modern retailing.

Buying commodities was not the main inducement that drew crowds to frequent the department stores that flourished in Korea during the 1930s and '40s. Rather, the 'retail palaces' provided an opportunity for the urban masses to participate in the public culture of spectacle that came to characterize the modern city. Dining out in these locations was part and parcel of the experience of being modern. Department stores allowed ordinary people to indulge temporarily in the fantasy of wealth and provided an opportunity to escape from the daily reality into a 'dream world' of commodities. This was particularly true for women, who had few reputable and justifiable ways to escape from the confinement of the domestic sphere.

Having said that, one must be conscious of the fact that terms such as 'ordinary people', 'urban masses' and 'crowds' need to be seen in a proper context. They refer to the bourgeois class of land-owners, entrepreneurs and urban professionals, rather than disowned farmers, coolies and factory girls. The department store was a destination for going out, which, as *Chosŏn Ilbo* advised its readers in December 1934, required from female visitors proper attire, hairstyling and make-up.[86] In 1936 a department store meal was worth a day's wage from an unskilled labourer, a ten-day supply of firewood for a family of five or a two-day supply of rice to feed them; it was more expensive than a pair of rubber-soled shoes.[87] When seen from this perspective, department store dining reveals a class dimension that vividly differentiates the crowds of department store customers from the rest of the Korean population.

This fact notwithstanding, these experiences, like many other aspects of colonial modernity, underline the complexity of the position that the Japanese assumed in colonial Korea – that of both an oppressor and a trendsetter. Moreover, the position of the Koreans was ambiguous as well, since the very survival of the trendsetter – the Japanese department stores – was in fact dependent on the patronage of their Korean clientele. The department stores in colonial Korea provided sites in which Japanese and Korean people – the colonized and the colonizers – could share the experience of being modern consumers seduced by things and fashions. Japanese and Koreans dined together in the grand dining halls of the department stores, and not infrequently the latter outnumbered the former.[88]

Considering the fact that the overwhelming majority of the Korean population lived in rural rather than urban areas, one might dismiss these experiences as marginal, since only a small fraction of

Koreans were able to familiarize themselves with the new culture of consumption. However, the relative importance of this incipient phase derives from the prominent role it acquired later. The major innovation of the department store was the creation of an entirely new environment for public leisure centred around shopping.

3
Industrializing Korean Taste

The 'Soul' of Korean Cuisine

The previous two chapters described developments closely tied to the experiences of the colonial period (1910–45), and more specifically to the period of roughly two decades that followed the liberalization of colonial rule from the 1920s onwards. These experiences functioned as the foundation of the transformations that the consumption practices of the Korean people underwent in the latter half of the century. As mentioned in the Introduction, one of the objectives of this volume is to demonstrate multiple connections between the colonial period and the post-1945 dietary developments on the peninsula. However, due to the lack of sources – and the reluctance of Japanese corporations to disclose their colonial past – it is often impossible to systematically document these connections. The case of the industrialization of soy sauce manufacture described in this chapter provides us with unique direct evidence of how colonialism permeated Korean cuisine. Further, what is striking about this aspect of the colonial legacy is that industrially produced soy sauce reached wide sections of the Korean population only several decades after Japanese rule had come to an end.

As mentioned briefly in the Introduction, fermented soyfoods, often referred to by their generic name, '*chang*', have played a central role in Korean cooking for centuries.[1] The three types of *chang* – soy sauce (*kanjang*), soybean paste (*toenjang*) and red chilli soybean paste (*koch'u-jang*) – are the very foundations of the Korean taste as we know it today, along with garlic, green onions and red chillies.[2] Although all three play an important role in providing Korean cuisine with its distinctive taste, the use of soy sauce in a wide range of dishes makes it quantitatively the most important type of *chang* in Korean cooking, the 'soul' of Korean cuisine.

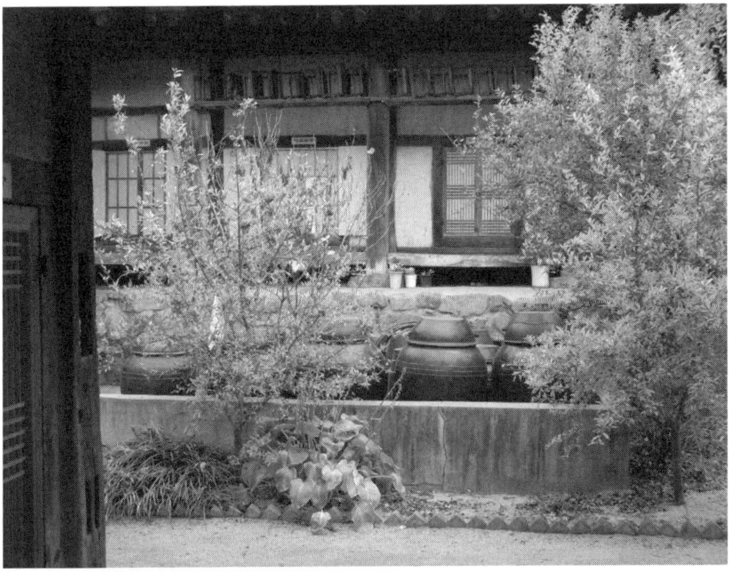

A traditional upper-class house in Hahoe Folk Village, near Andong, autumn 2003. Jars with soybean condiments maturing in the yard used to be a fixture of every household.

The manufacture and storage of *chang* were for centuries a key concern of women, who were responsible for the production and cooking of food.[3] Two major events that marked the passage of time in the Korean household were the pickling of *kimch'i* in late autumn and a range of activities related to the production of soybean pastes and sauces that stretched from winter to early summer. Compared to pickling *kimch'i*, the production of *chang* was a complicated affair, consisting of tasks that needed to be performed repeatedly at different times of the year.

First of all, the fermentation starter *meju* – dried lumps of fermented soybean mash – had to be manufactured. This took place in early winter, after the *kimch'i* pickling had been completed. The mash was made of soybeans soaked in water, boiled and shaped into lumps (bricks, discs, cones or balls) that were then dried in the sun for several days and left for up to two weeks in a warm place to ferment. Afterwards, *meju* chunks had to be left to dry in the sun yet again for several weeks. Great care was required when performing these chores – incorrect handling could mean being left without the most important ingredient for manufacturing *chang*. In early spring *meju* had to be immersed in brine in the ratio 2:4:1.2 (*meju*, water, salt), so that the salt concentration of the mash oscillated around 20 per cent. Charcoal and red chillies were added to the mixture; the former was supposed to remove impurities and the latter to sterilize the ingredients. The pulp was then placed in a large crock where amino acids and sugars formed by the breakdown of the soybeans exuded into the brine, and salt-tolerant yeasts had a chance to grow. After a few months the mixture acquired a dark brown colour and meaty flavour. At this stage *toenjang* and *kanjang* were not yet separated from each other. The liquid that was drained from the pulp, boiled and left to mature for 40 to 60 days, turned into the traditional Korean soy sauce, which could keep for several years. The mash that remained after the liquid had been drained was mixed with salt, packed tightly in a jar and then left to ferment in the sun for another month. The result was the classic Korean soybean paste.[4]

The making of soy sauce, soybean paste and chilli soybean paste was strictly a home affair for centuries. The preparation methods and flavour varied considerably, not only by region, but because each family had its own recipes handed down from generation to generation.[5] Because the taste of Korean dishes largely depends on the flavour of the *chang*, each household's home cooking acquired its distinctive flavour through the use of its sauces. With the industrialization of soy sauce manufacture, however, this distinction began to disappear.

By the late twentieth century, factory-made soy sauce had almost entirely replaced the home-brewed product in South Korea.[6] More importantly, it was not manufactured according to the traditional Korean method, but was based on the production processes that were introduced by the Japanese during the colonial period. Most Koreans do not realize that the soy sauce they consume on a daily basis is a product of the colonial experience. It seems neither useful nor possible to ascertain whether Koreans would have adhered faithfully to traditional processes right up to the present and never attempted to mass produce soy sauce if the Japanese had not shown them how. Identifying the implications of the industrialization of soy sauce production on Korean taste preferences, instead, will help us to comprehend the far-reaching, longstanding and unforeseen consequences of Japanese colonial rule.

Soy Sauce Manufacture in Japan

Inns and brothels were the first Japanese enterprises that opened in treaty ports to provide services to fellow countrymen who began to arrive in Korea after 1876. They were followed by small workshops producing consumer goods, from soap and tatami mats to sake and tofu.[7] City-dwellers, the majority of Japanese residents in Korea, relied on such workshops for their two major fermented soyfoods: *shōyu* (soy sauce, the equivalent of Korean *kanjang*) and miso (soybean paste, the equivalent of Korean *toenjang* and *koch'ujang*). This was particularly true of soy sauce, which had been commercialized in Japan since the seventeenth century.[8]

The classic Japanese procedure for brewing *shōyu* required whole-wheat grains to be parched and cracked and mixed with steamed soybeans. Spores of the mould *Aspergillus oryzae* were then added and the mixture incubated for three days. This process was comparable to *meju* making, but riskier and more labour-intensive, as the mixture had to be regularly tossed and the temperature of the incubation room constantly controlled. The next step was adding a brine solution and placing the acquired *moromi* mash in huge cedar casks that were then left to mature for several months. Again, the mash had to be stirred regularly

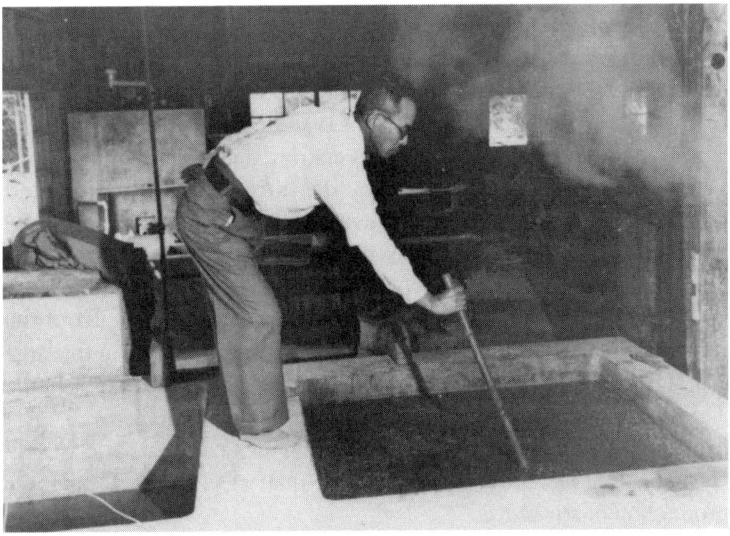

A Japanese soy sauce brewer checking the condition of a batch fermenting in a concrete vat, *c.* 1940s.

so fermentation would proceed evenly. When ready, the mash was pressed in cotton sacks under heavy weights to squeeze out the soy sauce – again more labour-intensive than the Korean method of draining the sauce, made possible by the more watery fermenting mixture in the manufacture of *kanjang*. The liquid was then pasteurized and transferred into wooden kegs.[9]

It is evident from this description that the Japanese method was much more labour-intensive than the Korean. The addition of wheat required a longer fermentation period, and it was not possible to use the lees remaining after the squeezing of the sauce for making soybean paste. All in all it was a costly method, hardly suitable for home manufacture. By the eighteenth century the best-quality *shōyu* was produced by commercial brewers clustered in large cities, while the rural population relied on homemade soybean paste for flavouring.[10]

The use of soy sauce by most farm households, which were largely self-sufficient in food, was restricted to special occasions such as festivals and weddings.[11] They purchased soy sauce from local brewers who offered it for as little as one-third of the price of the top city brands.[12] Wealthy farmers brewed soy sauce at home, an activity that continued well into the twentieth century, particularly in western Japan.[13] Travelling brewers also moved from area to area and supervised their customers' home brewing.[14] Nevertheless, rural *shōyu* could not approximate the quality of what was available in the cities.

Propelled by urbanization and rising living standards following the 1894–5 Sino-Japanese War, the demand for classic top brands of soy sauce such as Kikkōman, Yamasa and Higeta increased steadily. To meet this demand, leading brewers initiated wide-ranging innovations. Capacity was enhanced by the introduction of year-round production, modern machinery and new brewing methods based on scientific research.[15] Production, organization and management were modernized, unleashing mergers, incorporations and takeovers among soy sauce producers. The number of manufacturers diminished and the market share of the largest firms grew rapidly, at first mainly in the large cities. Between 1923 and 1931 the share of the top three brands in the Tokyo market increased from 45.9 to 67.6 per cent.[16] The five largest firms managed to strengthen their position on a national scale as well. By 1937 they accounted for nearly one-quarter of the total Japanese production of soy sauce.[17]

Before the 1920s the Japanese soy sauce industry had a two-tier structure: large manufacturers controlled the market in the big cities, and small- and medium-scale manufacturers targeted towns and villages.[18] When the economic boom triggered by the First World War began to show signs of slowing, the leading manufacturers turned to the rural market. While the top city brands did not emerge as national brands until the 1960s, the large manufacturers' shift to local markets forced smaller brewers to focus on low-cost *shōyu* and to increasingly rely on the second pressing of the sauce (*bansui*) and synthetic soy sauce.[19]

The introduction of amino acid liquid (*aminosan eki*), in English known as hydrolysed vegetable protein (HVP), revolutionized the industry. Soybeans were first hydrolysed through heating with 18 per cent hydrochloric acid for eight to twelve hours and then neutralized with sodium carbonate. The resulting product was a clear dark-brown liquid which was usually mixed with caramel colouring, corn syrup, salt and water so as to resemble the original soy sauce. This synthetic product could practically be made in a day. Its taste, however, was inferior to the fermented product and in practice most manufacturers mixed it with fermented soy sauce to achieve a balance between product quality and production efficiency.[20]

Synthetic soy sauce was developed as a by-product in the production of monosodium glutamate. The leading producer of MSG, the Suzuki Chemical Company, had been experimenting with HVP since the late 1920s.[21] After 1929, when Suzuki's patent on the manufacture of MSG expired, many companies began producing monosodium glutamate and HVP.[22] Nihon Chisso Hiryō (Japan Nitrogenous Fertilizers, Nitchitsu for short) released an artificial soy sauce named Soyament or Soyamint in 1931, which was marketed in the U.S.[23] Despite Nitchitsu's efforts, the Suzuki Chemical Company emerged as the leading producer of HVP and began selling it to small-scale brewers in 1933.[24] Mixed with fermented *shōyu*, HVP liquid performed well as a low-cost substitute for the classic flavouring.[25] Still, before the 1940s, it dominated only the lowest rungs of the market: fermented soy sauce prevailed.

The outbreak of the Sino-Japanese War in 1937 propelled chemical soy sauce from the periphery to the centre. Faced with increasingly severe resource shortages, Japanese manufacturers using conventional methods could no longer meet civilian demand and ensure supply for the rapidly expanding Japanese army. In 1941 a government decree ordered all soy sauce producers to rely on the synthetic product.[26] The Amino Acid Control Association was set up in the same year, following similar organizations that coordinated each branch of industry in the wartime economy.[27]

The Suzuki Chemical Company responded to the new regulations by establishing Takara Shōyu Industries (Takara Shōyu Kōgyō), a joint venture with Chōshi Shōyu.[28] At its peak the company manufactured 5.5 million litres of chemical soy sauce annually by mixing Suzuki's HVP liquid with soy sauce brewed by Chōshi at an 80:20 ratio. This ratio was particularly high; most producers used its opposite, 80 per cent brewed soy sauce and 20 per cent HVP.[29] Suzuki's output of HVP liquid was much larger. When production peaked in 1942, the company was manufacturing over 25 million litres a year (see p. 182, Chart 1), but production declined after 1942 as the wartime government prioritized the manufacture of aluminium.[30]

Given the increasing shortage of resources, further modifications in soy sauce manufacture were implemented. In 1943 the research laboratory of Noda Shōyu, a cartel of soy producers, developed a new method of soy sauce production which involved partially hydrolysing copra lees (the remains of coconut after squeezing out the oil) with hydrochloric acid, adding mould spores to the mixture and letting it ferment for one to two months. The expansion of the Japanese Empire into Southeast Asia secured supplies of the new ingredient. In 1948 Noda Shōyu perfected this semi-fermenting method, which was made available to other producers via the Japan Soy Sauce Association.[31]

Chemical soy sauce (a mixture of fermented soy sauce with HVP in varying ratios) and the semi-fermented product described above continued to dominate the soy sauce market in Japan until the 1960s. The Japanese Agricultural Standard (JAS) for soy sauce introduced in 1963 still allowed fermented *shōyu* to contain up to 80 per cent HVP.[32] The turning point came seven years later when Kikkoman Co. (formerly Noda Shōyu) decided to discontinue manufacture of semi-fermented soy sauce.[33] This decision was critical for the entire market since Kikkoman was its most powerful player. As Yokotsuka points out, Kikkoman's decision was informed by post-war technological advances that allowed for more efficient production of fermented soy sauce.[34] With the standard of living rising, the company saw new opportunities in the classic, brewed product. Today JAS does not allow the addition of HVP to first-class fermented soy sauce (*honjōzō shōyu*). In 1995 semi-fermented soy sauce and soy sauce containing HVP liquid constituted 17.8 and 5.6 per cent of the Japanese market share respectively.[35] These figures stood in sharp contrast to the situation in South Korea: as of 1993, 96.7 per cent of all soy sauce retailed in South Korea contained HVP liquid.[36]

The Japanese Soy Industry in Colonial Korea

Commercial soy sauce breweries appeared in Korea long before the changes described above took place in Japan. Yamamoto Soy Sauce Brewery was the first, opening a workshop in the port of Pusan in 1885 or 1886.[37] Similar small-scale enterprises followed in Wŏnsan, Inch'ŏn, Keijō and Chinnamp'o. Their number and geographical distribution grew steadily after 1905, when the Japanese flocked to the protectorate in search of business opportunities. By the 1920s approximately 100 soy sauce breweries were clustered in urban areas with large Japanese populations.[38]

The precise number of commercial soy sauce manufacturers in colonial Korea is difficult to determine. Many of them were transient affairs run on negligible capital, in business one season and out the next. Those that employed less than five workers were not listed in company registers; those that were listed were often combined with other businesses like money lending, the retailing of foodstuffs and real estate. If brewing was a sideline, records were generally lacking, as was the case with many alcohol breweries that also manufactured soy sauce. Finally, company registers published by different organizations in different years contradict each other; possibilities for human error in the records cannot be underestimated.

Data for the wartime period (1937–45) of 'planned economy' and controlled distribution of resources is much more reliable. Manufacturers acquired raw materials and distributed their products via a network of producers' cooperatives and control associations.[39] Operating outside this network was practically impossible.

The majority of breweries established before the 1930s were small-scale, often family businesses that depended on traditional Japanese methods and limited investment. Most employed no more than ten workers while their yearly output was less than 100,000 litres – a scale comparable to most breweries in Japan.[40] However, larger enterprises operated in the colony, too. In the early 1920s Yamane Shōyu Brewery in Pusan produced over 300,000 litres of soy sauce a year. The brewery was owned by Yamane Takichi, who had come to Korea in 1901 from Yamaguchi Prefecture in western Japan. After trying various jobs, he began in the soy sauce and miso business in 1908. Another successful Pusan soy sauce brewer was Yoshii Shōji, who came to Korea in 1893 from Ōita Prefecture in northern Kyushu and began work at a company called Chūshun Shōten.[41] Fifteen years later he was responsible for managing the brewing branch of the business.[42]

The largest brewery in the colony was the Japan Soy Sauce Company (Nihon Shōyu Kabushiki Kaisha) in Inch'ŏn. Established in 1905 as a subsidiary of Noda Shōyu, it came under the management of Okuda Teijirō, one of the era's most influential entrepreneurs; due to organizational changes within the parent company, in 1925 Nihon Shōyu officially became a Korean branch of Noda Shōyu.[43] In the early 1920s the Inch'ŏn factory was producing approximately 1 million litres a year, but by 1930 output had doubled, making it comparable to the largest factories in Japan.[44]

Top Japanese brands such as Kikkōman, Yamasa and Kihaku were highly valued by Japanese expatriates and imported in large quantities.[45] By establishing a subsidiary in Korea, Noda Shōyu had gained a head start over its competitors. Dominant in the Korean market, it worked on expanding sales in China, where it opened a sales office in Mukden (today's Shenyang) in 1918.[46] After the Manchurian Incident in 1931 and increased prospects for a large Japanese presence (and soy sauce demand) on the continent, similar trends could be observed in the soy sauce industries of colonial Korea and Japan: investment in facilities for mass production and market share consolidation. Existing breweries expanded operations or merged into larger enterprises. Still, large ventures were exceptional among soy sauce breweries in colonial Korea. In 1936 the Keijō Chamber of Commerce counted among manufacturers of soy sauce, miso and pickles only one factory that employed more than 200 workers, one that employed up to 30 workers, three with up to ten employees and eight with less than five.[47] The spectacular change was brought about by the outbreak of the Sino-Japanese War in 1937. According to one estimate, 276 factories were in operation by the end of 1942.[48] Forty new factories sprung up in 1941 and 1942 alone (see p. 176, Table III), while production more than doubled between 1939 and 1942, from 22,698,000 to 51,344,000 litres.[49]

The industry was concentrated in four provinces. Two provinces in southern Korea had a longstanding tradition of soy brewing: South Kyŏngsang's 53 factories in 1942 produced 8,890,000 litres (17 per cent of total production), and Kyŏnggi's 46 factories, 14,936,000 litres (29 per cent). Two other productive areas were located in northern Korea. South P'yŏngan Province counted only 16 factories, but produced 7,729,000 litres (15 per cent), nearly as much as the 53 factories in South Kyŏngsang. North Hamgyŏng Province in the northeast corner of the country

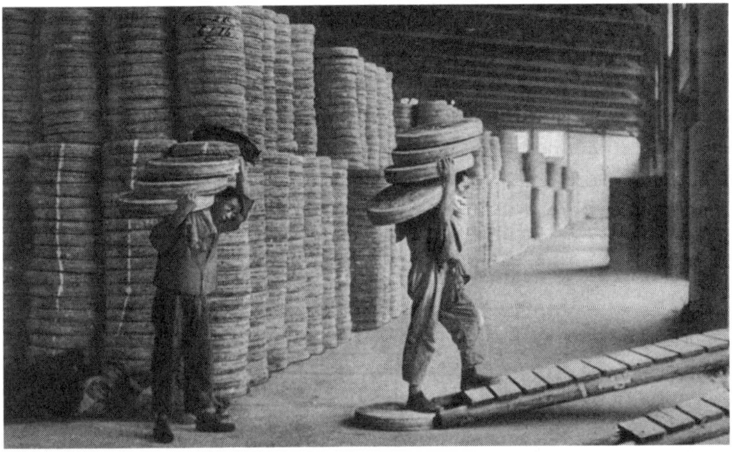

Manchurian labourers transporting cartwheel-shaped discs of soybean cake, made from mechanically pressing out the oil from soybeans, *c.* 1930s. This by-product of traditional Chinese soybean oil presses found a new application in HVP manufacture.

had 31 factories which together produced 5,399,000 litres (10 per cent). This extremely high volume of production implies that many factories in South P'yŏngan were using the new, synthetic technology (see p. 182, Chart II). This surmise is supported by additional evidence. From the late 1920s onwards, *shōyu* brewers in Japan increasingly relied on soybeans from Korea and Manchuria.[50] However, export of Korean soybeans to Japan declined after 1938, and was discontinued entirely after 1942.[51] Meanwhile, the amount of soybeans utilized in soy sauce manufacture in Korea drastically increased between 1939 and 1941 by 35 per cent (from 34,640 to 46,978 *koku*). Moreover, the use of soybean cake – never utilized in the Korean soy sauce industry before 1940 – rose from around 2,000 tonnes in 1940 to 2,870 tonnes the following year, indicating a growing reliance on HVP in manufacturing.[52]

Chōsen Chisso – a Korean subsidiary of Nitchitsu – began producing chemical soy sauce in 1940. Chōsen Chisso was the most prominent conglomerate operating in Korea, by 1945 accounting for some 35 per cent of the total Japanese direct investment and monopolizing the fertilizer, mining, synthetic fuel and electric power industries.[53] Soy sauce manufacture took place in the vicinity of Hŭngnam in northern Korea, in a complex chemical plant that combined the manufacture of chemical fertilizers, soap and margarine with dynamite, acetone and aluminium.[54] Nitchitsu began the chemical processing of soybeans in 1935 with the establishment of Soybean Chemical Industries

(Daizu Kagaku Kōgyō Kabushiki Kaisha) in Hŭngnam. The story goes that Noguchi Jun, the man behind the company, became interested in soybeans after he noticed that much of Manchuria's crop was being exported to Germany for use in chemical manufacture.[55] In 1936 a new brand of MSG named Asahi Aji and produced by Soybean Chemical Industries – the only competitor of the leading brand, Ajinomoto, on the Korean market – went on sale, while its chemical soy sauce followed in 1940.[56] According to the records of the Industrial Bureau of the Government-General from 1941, three other soy sauce manufacturers located in the Hŭngnam-Hamhŭng industrial complex also produced chemical soy sauce.[57]

The soy sauce industry in Korea expanded rapidly under the wartime economy; proximity to abundant supplies of soybeans and transportation routes favoured efficient, large-scale manufacture.[58] The branching out of leading Japanese soy sauce manufacturers into Manchuria and Korea intensified in the late 1930s and early '40s. Noda Shōyu began by transforming its sales office in Mukden into Manshū Noda Shōyu.[59] By 1945 Noda Shōyu operated nine soy sauce and soybean factories outside Japan: two in Korea, three in China and four in Southeast Asia.[60] Yamasa Shōyu followed in 1940 with Manshū Yamasa Company and two factories in Changchun in Northern Korea. Also in 1940, Marukin Shōyu opened a brewery in Liaoyang (south of Shenyang), and two years later, one in Masan, north of Pusan.[61]

With the exception of the wartime expansion of leading Japanese brewing firms, the overwhelming majority of soy sauce factories in colonial Korea were set up and managed by Japanese businessmen already settled in the colony. As I mentioned in chapter One, from the 1920s onwards Korean landlords and wealthy merchants slowly began to participate in Korea's industrialization by investing in small-scale food-processing factories such as rice mills. The overall share of Korean entrepreneurs, however, remained low throughout the colonial period, a meagre 6 per cent at the end of 1940.[62] I managed to locate fifteen soy-sauce-brewing enterprises that were owned (and run) by Koreans, sometimes jointly with Japanese.[63] The frequency with which Japanese-owned soy sauce breweries employed Korean managers is difficult to assess. I was able to locate Yi Sang-yŏn, a representative of Nagata Shōten in Shinŭiju (Shingishū), Kim Wan-sŏk, a representative of Sasaki Jōzōjō in Ch'ŏngjin (Seishin), Kim Sun-jak, a representative of Yamatsuru Jōzōjō Co. in Keijō and Kim Hong-gu, a factory manager for Yamada Shōyu in Masan.[64]

Last but not least, Japanese soy sauce breweries in Korea made extensive use of Korean labour. In 1924 a total of 627 workers were employed in Japanese-run soy sauce breweries in Korea, 430 of them (68 per cent) Korean nationals.[65] Twelve years later the Keijō Chamber of Commerce listed 120 Korean men and 30 women who were employed by soy sauce, miso and pickle factories operating in the city.[66] The number of workers increased as new factories mushroomed in the late 1930s and '40s; it seems plausible that some of the employed Koreans became proficient in the manufacture of Japanese-style soy sauce.

The primary consumers of Korean-made *shōyu* were the Japanese in Korea and, from the 1920s, Japanese communities in China. Due to lower production costs, *shōyu* made in Korea was able to compete with Japanese products, and was exported in small quantities to the homeland.[67] After 1937 the build-up of the Japanese armed forces on the continent turned Japanese troops into important consumers of Korean *shōyu*. Sales to the military by the Korean branch of Noda Shōyu increased steadily, oscillating between one-third and one-half of the total. The records of the Manshū Yamasa Company indicate that 40 per cent of their production was contracted by the military.[68]

Korean civilians also began to consume industrially produced Japanese soy sauce – an estimated 15 per cent of the population in 1942.[69] Although eagerness by some upper- and middle-class Koreans to imitate Japanese consumption practices may have been an incentive, it is more probable that wartime food shortages forced the situation. As the salt and soybeans necessary for the home manufacture of *kanjang* grew difficult to obtain, urban Koreans became increasingly dependent on industrially produced soy.

The Soy Sauce Industry in South Korea

By the end of 1946 most of the Japanese residents in Korea had been repatriated; the fate of the many enterprises they left behind often remained unknown. Many of them, however, made a lasting imprint on postcolonial Korea.[70] This was also the case with soy sauce breweries; in his report of 1949 for the U.S. Department of Agriculture, Allan K. Smith writes that 'in addition to homemade soy sauce, a supply is also available from many small factories making it. There are more than 10 plants in Seoul, the capital city.'[71] The predecessor of today's market leader, Sempio Foods Company (Saemp'yo Sikp'um Chusik Hoesa), was one of these ten plants.

The enemy property privatization bill, passed by the South Korean Congress in December 1949, began to be implemented in June the following year. Due to the outbreak of the Korean War and the need to stabilize the economy, a pre-emptive rights-based privatization method became dominant in this process.[72] Priority was given to those who had previously managed the Japanese enterprises, either under Japanese rule or during the U.S. military rule that followed Japan's capitulation in August 1945. It was believed that the former managerial staff would be able to restore production swiftly, something a public auction of the property could not guarantee. Consequently many Japanese enterprises ended up in the hands of those Korean managers who had run them during the colonial period.

The oldest surviving soy sauce manufacturer in South Korea today – the Monggo Food Company (Monggo Sikp'um Kong'ŏp Chusik Hoesa) – is a typical example. The brewery was established in Masan (South Kyŏngsang province) in 1905 as Yamada Shōyu. In December 1945 it was taken over by Kim Hong-gu, the factory's manager since 1935, and renamed the Monggo Soy Sauce Industry Company (Monggo Changyu Kong'ŏpsa) after the famous Monggo well that supplied water to the brewery.[73]

The fate of another Japanese company, which to this very day successfully operates in South Korea under the name Sempio Foods, took a slightly different turn. For over two decades since its establishment in 1916, the enterprise had been known as the Mitsuya Vinegar Brewery (Mitsuya Su Jōzōjō), embarking on soy sauce production some time between 1939 and 1941.[74] At the end of 1945 the management of the firm was transferred from the Japanese manager Ueyama Nakajirō to the American authorities. In July 1946 the management committee of twenty former employees was granted the right to continue production. The committee convinced Pak Kyu-hoe to take the responsibility of becoming the first director of this new business venture. Pak was a North Korean businessman who had during the colonial period worked for the (presumably Japanese) Wŏnsan Finance Corporation and South Korean Produce Co. After 1945 he headed south in search of new business opportunities.[75]

Information on the early post-liberation days of the two other soy sauce breweries that have survived to the present day is even less precise. It is not known which of the colonial breweries in Sunch'ŏn, South Chŏlla Province, formed the foundation of the Kim Bang Soy Sauce Factory (Kim Bang Changyu Kongjang), which was established in

August 1945 by a woman named Kim Bang. The feminine touch of the founder was eminently present in the branding of its soy sauce – the 'flower brand' (*kopp'yo*) derived from the ideogram of Ms Kim's first name. In 1979 the company was renamed Meil Foods Co. (Maeil Sikp'um Kong'ŏp Chusik Hoesa); it still operates successfully today.[76]

We know even less about Taech'ang Soyfoods Company (Taech'-ang Changyusa), set up in 1948 in Taejŏn, North Ch'ungch'ŏng Province, by Song Hŭi-baek. We may only presume that he took over one of the colonial factories that had been left in the city. In 1958 the firm was designated a contractor for the Republic of Korea Army and ten years later renamed Jinmi Foods Co. (Chinmi Sikp'um Chusik Hoesa).

These are four soy sauce manufacturers that stem directly from Japanese colonial breweries and still operate in South Korea successfully today, more than half a century after the end of colonial rule. If we consider that 131 industrial soy sauce manufacturers were operating in the Republic of Korea as of 1963, it seems plausible to surmise that many more colonial breweries must have been taken over,[77] especially if one considers that their geographical distribution very much resembled that of the colonial period (see p. 177, Table IV). Like their colonial predecessors before the wartime leap, most of these factories were very vulnerable – small, with limited distribution channels and negligible capital. Although very few single soy sauce breweries survived until the present day, the industry as such grew stronger. The number of soy sauce factories dropped below 100 only in the mid-1980s, due to the consolidation of the market, and remained stable, currently oscillating around 80.[78]

It is difficult to trace information concerning the pioneering days of South Korean soy sauce breweries. One aspect remains certain, however: that they utilized the Japanese method of manufacture and, like their Japanese counterparts at the time, relied heavily on HVP. But while the 1970s marked the beginning of the end of the era of chemical soy sauce in Japan, a similar trend did not emerge in South Korea until the 1990s. Between 1993 and 1997 sales of so-called 'mixed soy sauce' (*honhap kanjang*) – a mixture of fermented Japanese-style soy sauce and HVP liquid in varying concentrations – dropped from 75.6 to 69 per cent of all soy sauce retailed in South Korea.[79] Manufacturers predict that the South Korean soy sauce industry will move away from HVP in the near future. Yet, as in Japan, it was precisely this substance that determined the industry's survival after 1945.

Creating the consumer market for industrial soy sauce in Korea during the immediate post-liberation period proved more difficult than continuing production. As Japanese soldiers and civilians left the peninsula, pioneering enterprises had to rely on Korean consumers who, as we observed earlier, began to rely on industrial soy sauce because of the wartime shortage of resources. The demand from Koreans whose home production had been disturbed by war remained crucial during the 1950s, and was later largely sustained by rural-to-urban migration. The fledgling industry profited most from orders from the newly formed Republic of Korea Army, as was the case with other branches of the Korean food-processing industry.[80] Military demand increased tremendously after the outbreak of the Korean War (1950–53), and many breweries relocated production to the southeastern corner of the peninsula, which was spared from North Korean invasion. The war's displacement of people (see chapter Four) – from their homes and their homemade *kanjang* – also aided the sale of industrial soy sauce.

Generally speaking, it was necessity rather than choice that compelled Koreans during the first decade of independence to consume industrial soy sauce. Commonly known as *wae kanjang* (Japanese soy sauce), the factory-made product was regarded as inferior and clearly distinguished from the homemade product, which continued to be referred to simply as *kanjang* (soy sauce). Slowly but surely, however, factory-made soy sauce came to signify a modern urban lifestyle. The growing consumption of industrial soy sauce went hand in hand with South Korea's urbanization: in 1966 city-dwellers comprised merely 33 per cent of the population, a figure that had doubled only twenty years later. By the end of the twentieth century nearly 80 per cent of South Koreans lived in urban areas, while nearly 50 per cent resided in large cities with a population of more than 1 million.[81]

Today the term *wae kanjang*, used a few decades ago to refer to factory-made soy sauce, has fallen from use; industrial soy sauce (fermented or chemical) is now simply called *kanjang*. It has turned into an ordinary component of the daily existence of most (South) Koreans. Most consumers do not realize that in every bottle of soy sauce they purchase resides the invisible legacy of Japanese colonial rule.

MSG and Korean Cuisine

It seems obvious that the reliance on Japanese methods for the commercial manufacture of soy sauce in South Korea was determined by pragmatism: the methods were more suitable for large-scale production than the traditional Korean approach. This is yet another example of the colonial experience being a 'silent companion' to Korea's postcolonial development.[82] As Sidney Mintz convincingly argued in his study of sugar, production has a profound effect on consumption: what quantities of food are made available, when, and for how much, affect food choices and may have a lasting impact on consumption patterns.[83] The implications of the industrialization of soy sauce manufacture in Korea do not concern consumption patterns as such, but had a powerful impact on flavour. As more and more (South) Koreans today rely on industrially produced soy sauce, differences in taste that once marked the cooking of different regions have disappeared. Restaurants are almost entirely dependent on industrial soy, while the food-processing industry utilizes it extensively in a variety of products (see chapter Five). Thus the gradual shift from homemade to factory-made *kanjang* has brought about the *nationalization* of taste, making the flavour of Korean food uniform. As the last section of this chapter will demonstrate, however, soy sauce was not the only factor in the process of the standardization of taste in (South) Korea – a factor that was also of Japanese origin.

The early 1950s witnessed the first printed advertisements for factory-made *kanjang* targeted at urban consumers.[84] They suggestively linked the new product to modern living, represented by the rhetoric of industrial production, and convenience and efficiency in the kitchen. The Samsi Soy Sauce Brewery was particularly successful in cultivating this image. One of its strategies was to directly capitalize on the popularity of MSG by claiming that the use of this condiment was unnecessary when one flavoured one's food with Sempio-brand soy sauce.[85]

As mentioned earlier, synthetic soy sauce was developed in the 1920s as a by-product in the production of monosodium glutamate (MSG). MSG was an invention of a Japanese chemist, Ikeda Kikunae (1864–1936), and was patented in 1909 by the Suzuki Chemical Company under the brand name Ajinomoto (literally 'essence of taste').[86] The brand name soon acquired the generic meaning of MSG. Japanese soy sauce brewers and restaurateurs rejected the product, so the company's main initial target in Japan was enlightened bourgeois housewives who sought to manage their kitchens according to the principles of hygiene and nutritional science. In contrast, in Taiwan food vendors quickly embraced the flavour enhancer, and by the 1920s Ajinomoto was widely used in the colony by all social classes. 'It has established itself', Jordan Sand explains,

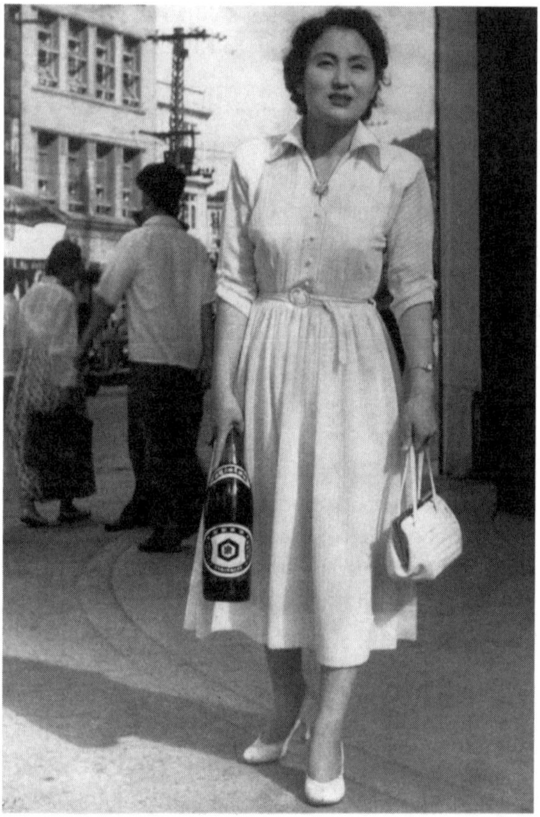

An advertisement for Sempio-brand soy sauce, 1958.

> as a cheap and commonplace part of the diet, without the experts' seals of approval, the rhetoric of hygiene and efficiency and the connotation of modern living that had been important to Ajinomoto's propagation in Japan.[87]

The sales of MSG in China suffered from anti-Japanese sentiments. Ajinomoto became a symbol of Japanese imperialism, an important weapon of Chinese manufacturers who fought for their share of the market. The largest one, Tian Chu ('Heavenly Kitchen'), consciously imitated Ajinomoto's packaging and advertising in its 'Buddha's Hand' (*foshou*) brand, but emphasized the fact that it was a domestic product.[88]

The Suzuki Chemical Company began to sell Ajinomoto in Korea in 1910, but exclusively targeted the Japanese community. Serious measures towards marketing the product among Korean consumers were undertaken after the establishment of the Keijō office in 1931. This year marked the saturation of urban markets in the Japanese home islands, prompting the management of Suzuki Chemicals to concentrate on promoting the product in rural areas, the colonies and other overseas markets. Promotional activities in Korea included setting up advertising lanterns and neon signs, placing advertisements in Korean-language newspapers and magazines, and distributing sample bottles at grocery stores, in restaurants and at markets.[89]

Sales of Ajinomoto in Korea nearly doubled between 1933 and 1936, reaching a peak of nearly 270 tonnes two years later.[90] If we consider that a domestic brand of MSG (Asahi Aji) manufactured by a subsidiary of the Nitchitsu concern in North Korea went on sale in 1936, the colonization of the Korean taste by MSG became irreversible. It is important to note that Ajinomoto-brand MSG was widely used to flavour Korean food. For example, it was used extensively to enhance the taste of the meat-based stock of vendors selling 'cold noodles' (*naengmyŏn*) and beef soup (*sŏllŏngt'ang*).[91]

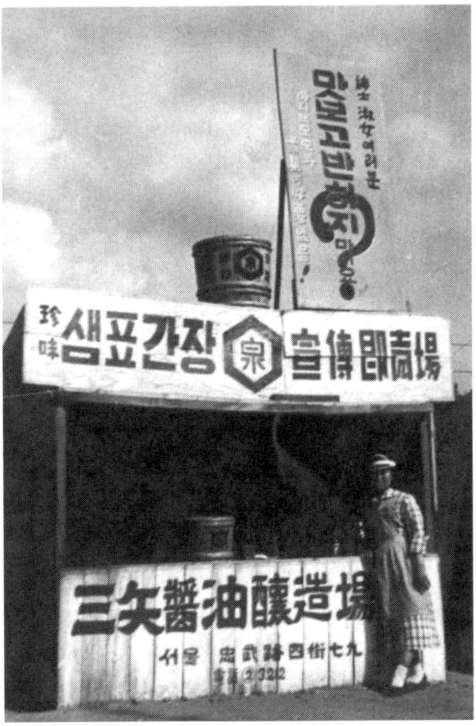

A stand advertising Sempio-brand soy sauce, 1954.

The rhetoric of modernity, similar to that in Japan, was critical in the construction of Ajinomoto's progressive image in the colony. Phrases such as 'the seasoning of civilization', 'seasoning of the new era' and 'worldwide seasoning' were often used in advertisements, and promotional campaigns were conducted at schools and exhibitions.[92] As Ajinomoto was increasingly used in private and professional kitchens throughout Korea, the taste buds of its consumers became more and more accustomed to its flavour.

Since after 1939 chemical soy sauce and war chemicals took priority in the production strategies of both manufacturers of MSG – the Suzuki Chemical Company and Soybean Chemical Industries – Korean consumers were entirely deprived of the seasoning they had so ardently embraced. Ajinomoto circulated in small quantities on the black market, but it was only in the mid-1950s that Koreans were able to produce their own MSG; Asahi Aji, manufactured by a subsidiary of the Nitchitsu concern in the mid-1930s, was a Japanese product. Moreover, poverty caused by the devastations of the Korean War (1950–53) meant that it took another decade before luxury products such as MSG became affordable to a wider range of the population.[93] Daesong Industry began to produce Mimiso in 1955, and a year later Donga Whaseong started manufacturing its Miwon, which soon became a leading brand of MSG in South Korea. In his analysis of the Korean history of MSG, Keun-Sik Jung argues that the 'embedded memory of Ajinomoto' in Miwon's name was essential for its commercial success.[94] Although the Chinese characters used in writing '*miwŏn*' and '*ajinomoto*' are not exactly the same, their meaning is identical: the 'essence' or 'origin' of 'taste'. 'In the social history of MSG in Korea,' Jung writes,

> the contradiction that lies in the process of transition from Ajinomoto to Miwon is what represents the dualism of colonial modernity. Ideologically, Ajinomoto was an object to be rejected as it symbolized Japanese colonization, but in the world of taste already embedded in the body, it was maintained as an unconscious inclination and desire.[95]

The claim of Samsi Brewery in its 1954 advert that the use of MSG was unnecessary when one flavoured one's dishes with Sempio-brand soy sauce (which contained HVP liquid) was by no means ungrounded. Due to the chemical composition of HVP liquid, its taste resembles the taste of naturally brewed soy sauce with MSG added to it.[96] Because Korean

An advertisement for Miwon-brand MSG, 1966.

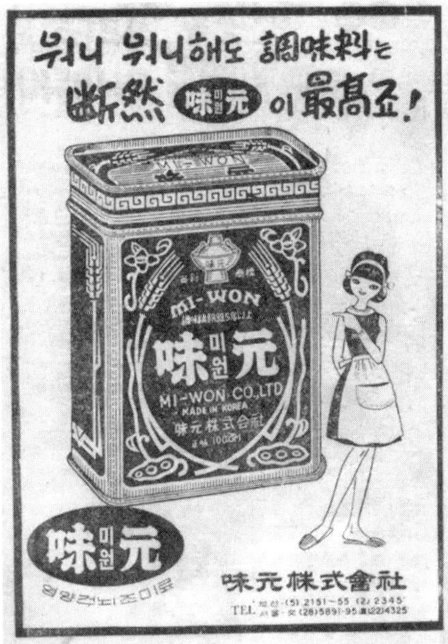

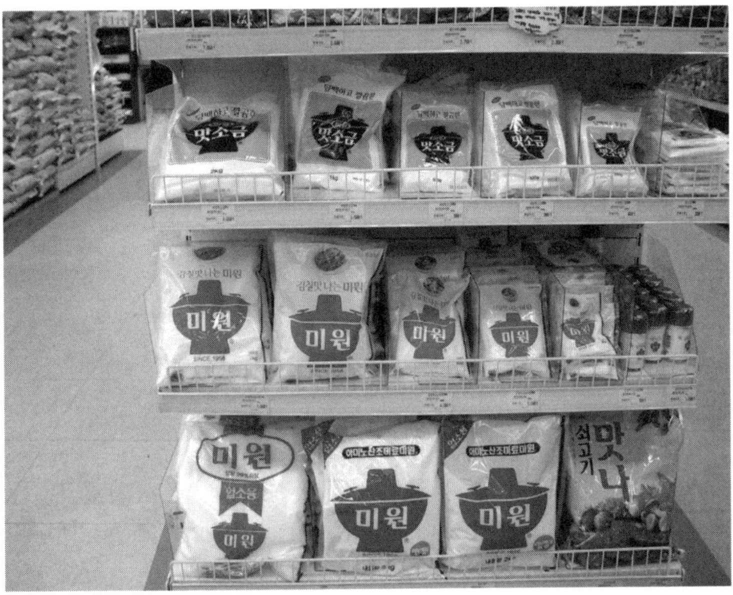

Various sizes of Miwon-brand MSG on sale in a South Korean supermarket, 2003.

consumers were already familiar with this taste at the time when they began to be targeted as potential consumers of factory-made soy sauce, we may speculate that the embedded memory of Ajinomoto played a role in the acceptance of industrial soy.

4
Wartime Food Management and Its Legacy

> Everyone received a full bowl of steaming rice, and I made some soft porridge for the baby. It was more than we had to eat at one time in many weeks. Our concave stomachs growled, but when the food was in our mouths we could not swallow it down. Our bellies were in shock. Even our fingers had forgotten how to use chopsticks. It was as if they had never held them before.[1]

Famine, disease and hunger are close accomplices of war, not infrequently begetting more victims than bombs and bullets. It has been estimated that more than half of the troops that the Japanese armed forces lost during the Second World War in the Pacific did not die on the battlefield, but perished due to malnutrition-related diseases and starvation.[2] Famine of a magnitude comparable to the one that hit northern Vietnam in the winter of 1945, wiping out an estimated 1.5 million people, did not take place on the Korean peninsula.[3] However, for the majority of the Korean population hunger constitutes one of the most powerful memories of the 1940s and '50s. It ranks among the most vivid reminders of the evils of Japanese colonial administration, the derisory mismanagement of the American occupying forces south of the 38th parallel, and the widespread looting of the northern half of the country by Russian forces. In public memory hunger symbolically marks the mid-twentieth century as the common experience of *all* Koreans, despite the fact that not everybody went hungry – for example, during the second half of the 1940s the agricultural population in general was better fed than it had been for years,[4] not to mention black-marketeers and other entrepreneurs who capitalized on the opportunities offered by the wartime and post-war chaos. Yet a normative connection that had developed over the decades between patriotism and suffering makes it difficult for any South Korean *not* to subscribe to the national allegory of hunger.[5]

There is no doubt that there was a shortage of food in Korea during the 1940s and '50s. The main purpose of this chapter is to chronicle how it unfolded, exacerbated by bad harvests, disastrous economic policies and wartime destruction. In the rapidly shifting political scene of mid-twentieth-century Korea, no regime in power at any given moment was able to solve the food shortage problem. Neither could they afford not to address this issue, since it had the potential to pose a threat to public order. Thus food was placed high on the agendas of all the governments that took charge of the Korean peninsula throughout the 1940s and '50s. Interestingly, but by no means surprisingly, successive regimes often chose to inherit measures that were already in place or resurrected ones that had worked before in order to keep the food supply stabilized. Multiple connections between pre- and post-1945, and pre- and post-1950, are clearly expressed in the ways in which authorities handled the 'hunger problem'.

Food management is a powerful example of the structural continuities between colonial and postcolonial Korea. An analysis of its role provides strong evidence that the Korean War was a critical factor in keeping alive the legacy of the measures implemented by the Japanese during the early 1940s.[6] The focus on food clearly contradicts the dominant historical narratives of modern Korea, which tends to delineate the year 1945 as the fundamental turning point in Korean history, downplaying any possibility of connection between pre- and post-1945 developments.

Before examining the details, we first need to grasp the turbulent developments that had occurred in the region since the outbreak of the Pacific War (1941–5). The Japanese attack on the United States naval base at Pearl Harbor on 7 December 1941 crippled American control over the Pacific, allowing for swift Japanese encroachment into Southeast Asia. By summer 1942 the Japanese controlled the Philippines, British Malaya, Hong Kong, Singapore, French Indo-China and the Dutch East Indies, along with their colonies of Taiwan, Korea and Manchukuo. At this point the Allied powers gradually began to recover supremacy in the Pacific. In anticipation of the possibility of Japanese defeat, the Allied leaders met in Cairo in November 1943, where the fate of Japan's colonial possessions was discussed for the first time. The idea of a joint trusteeship of Japan's former colonies by Allied powers was confirmed at the meetings at Yalta (4–11 February

1945) and Potsdam (17 July–2 August 1945), but no plan or timetable concerning the trajectory towards an independent Korea was considered in detail.[7] When, under the impact of the two atomic bombs dropped on Hiroshima and Nagasaki in the early days of August 1945, the Japanese signalled their intention to surrender, American strategists chose to limit the Russian involvement in Korea. Instead of a joint occupation, they hastily suggested a North–South division along the 38th parallel, which was silently accepted by the Soviet side. This was one of the many steps that proved to be of profound consequence for Korea's future.

The United States–Union of Soviet Socialist Republics Joint Commission met several times throughout 1946 and 1947 to discuss the possibility of the envisaged joint 'trusteeship' over a unified and independent Korea. However, as the Cold War took on a definitive shape in the spring of 1947, the tensions between the two zones of occupation on the Korean peninsula grew stronger. The establishment in 1948 of two separate Korean states – the Republic of Korea (ROK) in the South and the Democratic People's Republic of Korea (DPRK) in the North – ultimately led to a civil war commonly known as the Korean War (1950–53). Although the conflict broke out in the early hours of 25 June 1950 with a massive North Korean assault over the 38th parallel, historians agree that the formation of the separate states in the North and South two years earlier marked its actual beginning.[8] Halted with the armistice agreement of 27 July 1953, the Korean War never really 'ended': no peace treaty has been signed so far.[9]

The toll of war was heavy. As many as 3 million Koreans died, at least half of them civilians; 36,940 American and an estimated 900,000 Chinese soldiers lost their lives in combat. The scale of urban destruction was enormous, especially in the North, where Americans dropped more bombs than in the entire Pacific theatre during the Second World War.[10] But beyond that, the war scarred Koreans for generations. The division of occupation zones along the 38th parallel, hastily arranged in August 1945, divides the North and South to the present day, and is a vivid reminder that Korea was the place where the Cold War arrived first and where it never left.

This mid-century war-waging, intertwined with Japanese colonial rule, was one of the most powerful historical forces that not only left a footprint in history books but had a lasting impact on the daily life of the Korean population. In terms of diet, the impact of war was far more complex and contradictory than food shortages alone. The industrialization

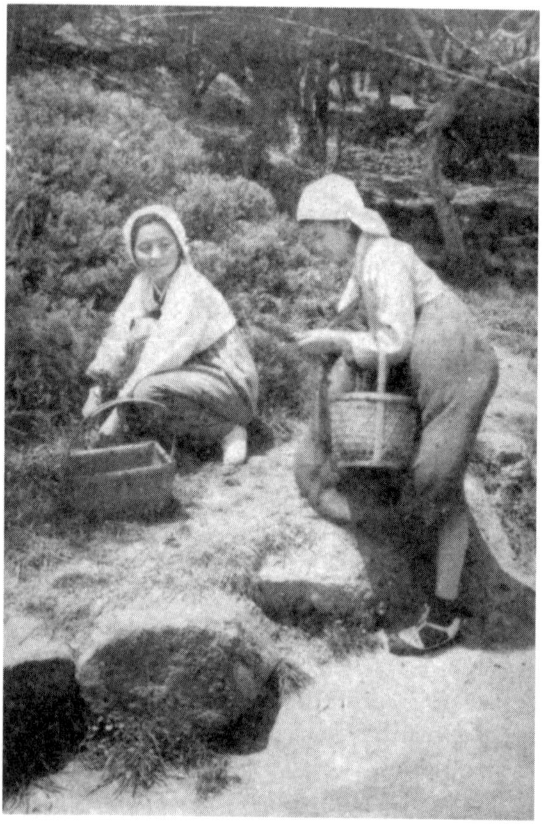

A Korean War-era postcard showing Korean women collecting wild greens to remedy food shortages.

of soy sauce manufacture described in the previous chapter, and the growth of the Korean food-processing industry addressed in chapter One, are examples of wartime influences on the Korean food system that complement conventional narratives of war-induced hunger and disease. As studies to date have indicated, wartime diets may serve as valuable sources of historical inquiry, revealing continuities that intricately connect the pre-war with the post-war.[11] The associations between the Sino-Japanese War and the Korean War, with the Cold War as a powerful shadow in the background, are striking. Collectively these three events not only shaped Korean lives during the 1940s and '50s, but transformed them for decades to come.

Within the immense body of research related to the Korean War there are surprisingly few descriptions of daily life. Generally speaking, scholarship on the Korean War has been rather proscriptive, examining

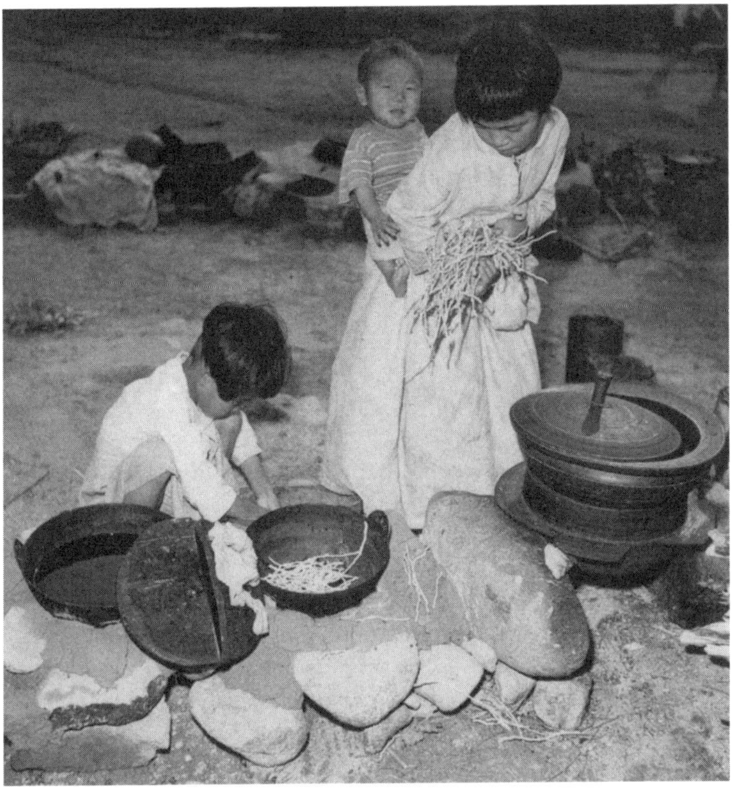

Children cooking a meal in the refugee camp at Yongdongpo, August 1951.

the conflict primarily from the angles of international politics, ideology and military strategy.[12] Similarly, the discourse on the effects of the Korean War on the Korean people has focused on the material devastation of the country and the disruption of identity caused by the division of the peninsula. Towards the end of the twentieth century, with the end of the Cold War and the democratization of South Korean domestic politics, increasing attention began to be paid to the structural, long-term social changes brought about by the war.[13] Still, due to lack of sources, it seems unlikely that the mundane, everyday experiences of Korean soldiers and civilians, the story of how 'life went on' despite the devastation, will ever be told. Photographic images and autobiographical fiction offer the best, however fragmented, narrative of the daily life of the Korean population during the turbulent years that preceded and followed the Korean War.[14]

Diaries and autobiographical novels provide us in the first place with an account of hardships as they have unfolded since the mid-1940s. Donald Chung's *The Three Day Promise: A Korean Soldier's Memoir*, written in English decades after the author settled in the United States, testifies that

> there was a severe shortage of food at this time, and we could only afford to eat rice once a day. Our country relatives helped us with offerings of beans and potatoes. We even ate the dried residue of yellow beans after the oil had been pressed out. Though such food was thought to be fit only as animal fodder, it had become a staple in the area even before the end of the war.[15]

Like the extract that opens this chapter, the quotation below describes the hardships of the refugees of the Korean War as they were recollected by the survivors, and passed on in their stories.

> We were assigned temporary housing in one of those large green military tents, contributions from the United Nations' relief organization . . . Each family received small weekly rations of rice and some stale vegetables, barely enough to sustain us. There was a chronic shortage of food and supplies. As a result, the menu rarely varied. It usually consisted of a bowlful of milky paste made from rice or the peeled skins of yellow soybeans. Sometimes I would dice weeds into our broth. For seven days a week, twice a day, that was our diet. The food would pass right through our systems. Watery it went in and watery it gushed out just a few hours later.[16]

On top of factual information, autobiographical literature also reveals the emotional responses of the Korean people to their shattered existence, with hunger featuring as a powerful icon of misery. A prime example is the novel *Who Ate Up All the Shinga?* by Park Wan-suh, which has sold over 1 million copies in South Korea since its publication in 1992.[17] It is a compelling story of a young girl coming of age in the midst of the historical turbulence of the 1940s and a bittersweet mother–daughter memoir, with food coming into the foreground as the situation deteriorated.

> The grain we now received was mixed with soy bean dregs that tasted awful . . . The smell of bean dregs was so disgusting . . . Mother and I ate the rice in which they'd been mixed, but of course a distinction existed here as well. At the top of our bowls, we seemed to have a similar proportion of dregs, but the deeper we went, the more dregs Mother's bowl held. I knew, but pretended not to notice because I despised them so much.[18]

Park describes her mother smuggling rice from thc countryside by stashing it in bundles of clothes and strapping it around her stomach.[19] In the final chapter hunger and malnutrition replace the mere disgust and inconvenience described earlier.

> Meanwhile, Sister-in-law had had an easy birth. She was crying quietly, her newborn second son at her side . . . Wrinkles were prominent on the malnourished infant's face, no bigger than a sweet potato. He was so tiny that he had slipped out from her womb without causing any labor pains.[20]

The novel ends at the point at which the protagonist takes flight from Seoul, scavenging on food abandoned by others.

> The clustered, vacant houses were now my prey. I was certain that each held at least a few handfuls of wheat flour, a small container or two of barley. I had accepted my gullet as my gang boss and no longer felt ashamed about it.[21]

Hunger features even more prominently in Hwang Sunwŏn's short story 'The Toad', set in Seoul shortly after the liberation and describing the misery of its protagonist Hyŏnse, a Korean refugee from North China.

> Hyŏnse sold his suit at the South Gate markets, bought the potatoes at the East Gate markets and put them in a sack, and started back to where his wife and children were. He was so hungry he couldn't help walking slouched over; he didn't even have the energy to wipe the sweat that was streaming from his forehead into his eyes and his mouth.

> Now it was the perspiration that was blurring his vision. All he could think of was steaming those damned potatoes and taking big bites out of them . . . blowing on them first if they were too hot . . . that light, powdery texture . . . but wait, just potatoes? . . . No, there had to be some cabbage-leaf soup to slurp, and he shouldn't eat the potatoes too fast . . . These thoughts had him drooling and swallowing the rest of the way home.[22]

The miserable conditions of Hyŏnse and his family are contrasted in the story with the relative well-being of the black-market entrepreneur Tugap, a former classmate Hyŏnse bumps into at a Seoul market. Tugap wears a 'well pressed and sleek suit' and has 'shiny oiled hair', but it is the smell of 'grilled beef and garlic, washed down with *soju*', the smell of Tugap's dinner the previous night, which works as a powerful literary tool in evoking the reader's repugnance.[23]

The 'voice' of the Korean people as disseminated in autobiographical literature is an important component in the exigent task of reconstructing the everyday life of mid-twentieth-century Koreans. Its role is particularly significant in the face of the shortage of other sources that document the transwar existence. While recognizing the value of this 'voice', caution is needed when utilizing it in historical research. To borrow the words of a prominent historian: 'Individuals construct and reconstruct their memories in much the same way as nations do their histories, creating what Borges called a "fictitious past" that they can live with.'[24]

The Japanese Management of Food Resources

The Japanese wartime government and military experts devoted a great deal of attention to the issue of food supply.[25] The National Mobilization Law (Kokka Sōdōin Hō) promulgated on 24 March 1938 provided the government with a legal basis for instituting wide-ranging reforms that aimed at the efficient use of food resources. Food shortages started to develop within the Japanese Empire shortly after the outbreak of the Second Sino-Japanese War in July 1937, and gradually price controls and rationing replaced the existing commercial channels of distribution. At the same time, a variety of measures aimed at educating civilians in the frugal preparation and consumption of food were disseminated.

The totalitarian character of the Japanese state bolstered the effectiveness of these reforms.[26]

The wartime management of food resources in Korea followed the pattern developed for Japan closely, although with a slight delay. The promulgation of the Korea Rice Market Company Ordinance (Chōsen Beikoku Shijō Kabushiki Kaisha Rei) in September 1939 was one of the first moves towards a government-controlled trade in grain.[27] The law effectively ended trade in rice based on the principles of the free market and replaced it by closed transactions between rice producers' cooperatives and rice dealers' associations in each prefecture. A quasi-governmental organization called the Japan Rice Company (Nihon Beikoku Kabushiki Kaisha) was from now on to handle Japanese rice imports from Korea and Taiwan.[28]

Because the Korean system of wartime food management closely mirrored the Japanese model, it is necessary briefly to explain the developments in Japan first. By February 1942, when the Foodstuffs Control Law (Shokuryō Kanri Hō) was promulgated, the Japanese authorities had introduced new methods and channels for the collection of grain that largely eliminated free-market mechanisms. The law facilitated putting control over the collection and distribution of staple foods entirely into the hands of semi-public corporations, so-called Shokuryō Eidan (Foodstuff Corporations). These corporations became responsible for the collection, storage and distribution/sale of staple rations to consumers, absorbing all merchants, wholesalers and cooperatives that had been involved in these processes thus far, including the Japan Rice Company established in 1939.[29]

The Foodstuffs Control Law of 1942 also introduced a uniform system of rationing staple foods. Before its promulgation, various forms of rationing and purchase-permit systems were already in place; these were managed by regional municipalities in Japan as well as in the colonies.[30] The new law replaced this variety with a uniform system, although in practice local differences in implementation continued. The Foodstuffs Control Law entitled every adult to a daily ration of approximately 330 grams (2.3 *gō*) of rice, with reduced rations for children and the elderly (see p. 177, Table v). Supplementary rations were available for labourers depending on their gender and the type of work they performed. At first the 'rice ration' was supposed to consist of rice alone, but due to shortages it soon had to be supplemented with wheat and barley. As the food supply situation deteriorated, the category was extended to include sweet and white potatoes, soybeans and other substitutes.

Moreover, the distributed quota tended to become increasingly lower than the quantity that people were entitled to buy according to their purchase permits. In the summer of 1945 the government was finally forced to reduce the daily staple food ration by nearly 30 grams, from 2.3 to 2.1 *gō*.[31]

Like the Korea Rice Market Company Ordinance, the Foodstuffs Control Law Enforcement Ordinance for Korea (Shokuryō Kanri Hō Chōsen Shikō Rei) was promulgated within a few months of the original law, on 26 June 1942. The document provided a legal basis for the implementation of most of the articles of the Foodstuffs Control Law, except for specific regulations concerning Food Corporations (paragraphs 16 to 18, paragraph 24 and article 1 of paragraph 19) and exports of rice, wheat and barley (paragraph 11). These were left to the discretion of the Government-General of Korea, as was the regulation of trade in other types of grain.[32] Korean rice exports to Japan continued, although falling dramatically after 1938 due to the reduced surplus (see p. 183, Chart III). This was caused by the combination of poor harvests and sizeable deliveries of rice to Japanese troops stationed in Korea and Manchuria. In 1940 roughly 150,000 tonnes of Korean rice was used for this purpose, more than twice the amount sent to Japan that year.[33]

On 9 August 1943 a separate Korea Food Management Law (Chōsen Shokuryō Kanri Rei) was instigated that replaced all earlier regulations related to the trade and distribution of grain in the colony, including the Enforcement Ordinance from the previous year.[34] Generally speaking, the law left the Government-General of Korea much freedom in determining the strategy of managing food resources, but stipulated the details concerning the establishment of the Korea Food Corporation (Chōsen Shokuryō Eidan) as an independent body responsible for the collection, storage, processing, distribution and rationing of grain in Korea. As in Japan, the corporation's main office was located in the capital, and branch offices were established in each prefecture to oversee the implementation of the new regulations.

Similarities in the wartime food management of Japan and Korea were not limited to monitoring producers and retailers alone. Near-identical mechanisms for controlling consumers were in place as well. Since rural consumers were practically self-sufficient in food supply, these mechanisms functioned primarily in urban areas. In Japan the task of coordinating the rationing of foodstuffs to consumers was from October 1942 entrusted to *tonarigumi* ('neighbourhood associations'). Composed of approximately ten households from each neighbourhood,

A poster from the travelling exhibition 'One Day from a Soldier's Life', organized by the colonial government to inspire Korean men to join the Imperial Japanese Army, 1940s.

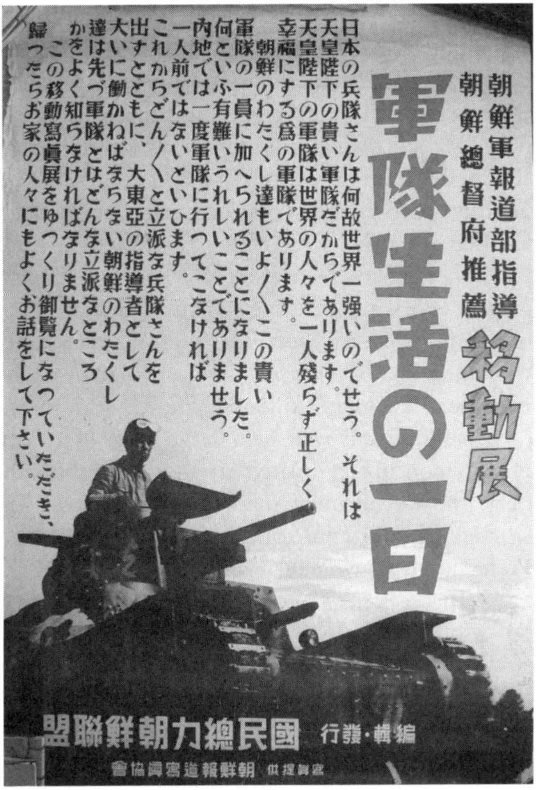
朝鮮軍報道部指導
朝鮮總督府推薦
移動展
軍隊生活の一日
日本の兵隊さんは何故世界一强いのでせう。それは
天皇陛下の貴い軍隊だからであります。
天皇陛下の軍隊は世界の人々を一人殘らず正しく
幸福にする爲の軍隊であります。
朝鮮のわたくし達もいよ／＼この貴い
軍隊の一員に加へられることになりました。
何といふ有難いうれしいことでありませう。
内地では一度軍隊に行つてこなければ
一人前ではないといひます。
これからどん／＼と立派な兵隊さんを
出すとともに、大東亞の指導者として
大いに働かねばならない朝鮮のわたくし
達は先づ軍隊とはどんな立派なところ
かをよく知らなければなりません。
この移動寫眞展をゆつくり御覧になつていただき、
歸つたらお家の人々にもよくお話をして下さい。
編輯・發行
國民總力朝鮮聯盟

the associations functioned as the de facto lowest level of municipal administration. Although set up with the original purpose of spiritual indoctrination within the framework of the Imperial Rule Assistance Association (Taisei Yokusankai), *tonarigumi* soon assumed a wide range of practical functions such as the certification of changes of address, collection of taxes, sale of war bonds and dissemination of government propaganda.[35] None of these activities, however, was as important as food distribution. The translation of *tonarigumi* as 'neighbourhood ration board' in the documentation of the Strategic Bombing Survey compiled by the U.S. Army Air Forces to evaluate the effectiveness of strategic bombing is perhaps the best example that testifies to this fact.[36]

A Korean version of *tonarigumi* – the so-called *aegukpan* or 'patriotic units' (translated by some scholars as 'neighbourhood patriotic units') – fulfilled exactly the same role in the colony.[37] By the end of 1939 over 370,000 of these units were functioning throughout Korea, the system being particularly well organized in and around the capital.[38] Composed of between ten and twenty households, *aegukpan* were organizationally integrated under the Korean Federation for Total Mobilization of National Spirit (Kokumin Seishin Sōdōin Chōsen Renmei), set up on 7 July 1938, and in October 1940 renamed as the Korean Federation for Total National Mobilization (Kokumin Sōryoku Chōsen Renmei). Replicating the model of the National Spiritual Mobilization Movement (Kokumin Seishin Sōdōin Undo) and its *tonarigumi* network in Japan, the *aegukpan* functioned as a civilian extension of colonial administration. Each unit was managed by a leader (*panjang*) who disseminated government directives received from the local administration to the member households. Monthly meetings (*pansanghoe*) of each 'patriotic unit' were held in the house of its leader on the tenth day of each month, coordinated in a uniform fashion through radio broadcasts. The overwhelming majority of 'patriotic unit' leaders in Korea were women. In 1942 approximately 70 per cent of *panjang* in Kyŏngsŏng Prefecture were women.[39]

The *aegukpan* system was in the first place designed to aid the policy of assimilation (*naisen ittai*, literally 'Japan Korea one body'), a strategy of cultural repression aimed at reshaping Koreans into loyal subjects of the Japanese empire. 'Patriotic units' played an active role in forcing Koreans to honour the Japanese state religion of Shinto, facilitated the mobilization of Korean labour and aided the conscription of Korean men into the Japanese armed forces.[40] However, like the case of *tonarigumi* in Japan, food rationing soon assumed a central place among *aegukpan* activities.[41] A Korean scholar, Hŏ Yŏng-nan, goes so far as to suggest that *aegukpan* should be renamed *paegŭppan* ('rationing units'), considering the pivotal role they fulfilled in the Korean rationing system.[42] By keeping track of the number of household members and forwarding this information to the municipal administration, *aegukpan* leaders played a vital role in the logistics of distributing foodstuffs to rationing points.[43] They also eased the work pressure of the municipal authorities by distributing rationing coupons, which were indispensable for the functioning of the rationing system. The seal of approval by *aegukpan* leaders had to be stamped on coupons before they could be used, reducing the risk of fraud. As in Japan, however, the abuse of this authority was widespread: rationed foodstuffs not infrequently ended up on the black market with the involvement of the very individuals who were supposed to prevent such illegal transactions.[44]

Rationing of food was not uniform throughout the colony. As was the case in Japan, the implementation of central regulations concerning staple food rations remained diverse, depending on the administrative capacities of each locality. Furthermore, the rationing of non-staple food items such as sugar, salt, meat and seafood was regulated independently by municipal authorities. In the colonial capital of Keijō, for example, by May 1943 the list of rationed commodities also included rice and other grains, wheat flour, sugar, salt, milk, alcoholic beverages, vegetable oil, starch, malt syrup, dried sardines, pollack roe, agar-agar, dried laver, beef and pork.[45]

Distribution of each item was handled by an association of the producers and retailers of each item and the purchasing procedure was quite complex. A family of up to four members was entitled to a ration of 50 *monme* (187.5 grams) of meat (either pork or beef) and a family of up to nine members 100 *monme* (375 grams). For larger households, 10 *monme* (37.5 grams) per family member was added to the daily ration. One family coupon was issued for each 'patriotic unit', each family being entitled to two meat coupons per month. The coupon could only be used on a specific date in a shop where the 'patriotic unit' was registered. If meat was sold out, the coupon could be used the following day, but only when the shop's seal was stamped on it (see also p. 184, Chart IV).[46] We may presume that by 1944–5 this neatly orchestrated procedure rarely took place, as the scarcity of goods had nurtured the growth of a black-market economy. In July 1945 the black-market price of rice was nearly 43 times its official wholesale price, that of barley 30 times and of wheat 20 times.[47]

The Food Situation in the South under the USAMGIK and ROK

The 24th Corps of the U.S. Tenth Army, under the command of General John Hodge, arrived at the port of Inch'ŏn on 8 September 1945. It was to function as the official ruling body of the southern half of the Korean peninsula until the formal inauguration of the Republic of Korea (ROK) on 15 August 1948. The only reason for selecting the 24th Corps, which had a long record of combat but no experience in civil affairs, for this task was simply that it could be sent to Korea at short notice, as it was recovering in Okinawa after a recent battle. The unit and its commander landed entirely unprepared for the complicated mission that awaited them. As the prominent historian of modern Korea

Michael Robinson bluntly put it, 'Hodge arrived in Korea with no translators, no area specialists, no background studies – fundamentally, no plan whatsoever.'[48]

Among the many problems that the United States Army Military Government in Korea (USAMGIK) was confronted with during its rule over the southern half of Korea, food security was a major one. To make things worse, it was largely of the USAMGIK's own making. On 5 October 1945 the newly installed government declared a free market in rice. According to an assessment of the situation provided in a report by the USAMGIK National Economic Board, the decision to liberalize the rice market was prompted by 'a near riot' that occurred southwest of Seoul in September 1945. 'Strict control of the rice market seemed inadvisable', explains the report, 'since the controls used by the Japanese backed by threats and punishment were to no avail and a flourishing black market had grown up.'[49] The assessment of the National Economic Board does not mention other reasons behind the American decision to introduce a free-market policy for rice in Korea. As Pu Mi-sŏn and other Korean researchers argue, the measure was intended in the first place to weaken the Committee for the Preparation of Korean Independence (Chosŏn Kŏnguk Chungi Wiwŏnhoe), a coalition group formed under the leadership of moderate leftist Yŏ Un-hyŏng (1885–1947) immediately after Japan's capitulation.[50] The committee's objective was to guarantee peace and order while in the meantime drawing up plans for an independent Korean government. Two days before the arrival of the Americans, on 6 September, it announced the formation of a People's Republic of Korea (PRK); its local branches, known under the name of People's Committees (Inmin Wiwŏnhoe), successfully assumed control over local levels of government, including the management of the local branches of the Korea Food Corporation that had been formed by the Japanese two years earlier.[51] Neither the Korean People's Republic nor the People's Committees were recognized by the U.S. authorities, who indiscriminately labelled them communists.[52]

Regardless of whether the reason behind the policy of decontrolling the grain market in October 1945 was a conscious strategy to fight communism or simply a human error that led from incorrectly assessing the situation, it proved fatal for the economy, resulting in an inflationary spiral that continued for years. In the first three months alone the price of rice skyrocketed from 32 won per 54-kg bag offered by the government in early October to 70 won by early November, and 160 won a month later.[53] As Bruce Cumings explains in his monumental work *The Origins of the Korean War*, 'the MG institutions of a free-market policy caused the bumper rice harvest in the fall of 1945 to evaporate virtually overnight, owing to the profiteering, speculation, hoarding, and increased rates of consumption of a population unaccustomed to the psychology of exchange on the open market.'[54] Cumings describes how private fortunes were made by police officials and provincial appointees of the newly established Military Government through the flourishing trade in rice, even involving smuggling rice to Japan.[55]

The full effects of the disastrous rice policies were not felt until the rice harvest of 1946. Since the rice collection programme of 1946 was considered by the Americans 'to be one of the most important, if not *the* most important means of helping to stabilize the economy, ease the acute food situation, and stem the continuing inflationary spiral in Korea',[56] they decided to revive the brutal methods of rice collection that had been practised by the Japanese authorities. Largely due to the association with Japanese colonialism, the recycled strategy failed, leading

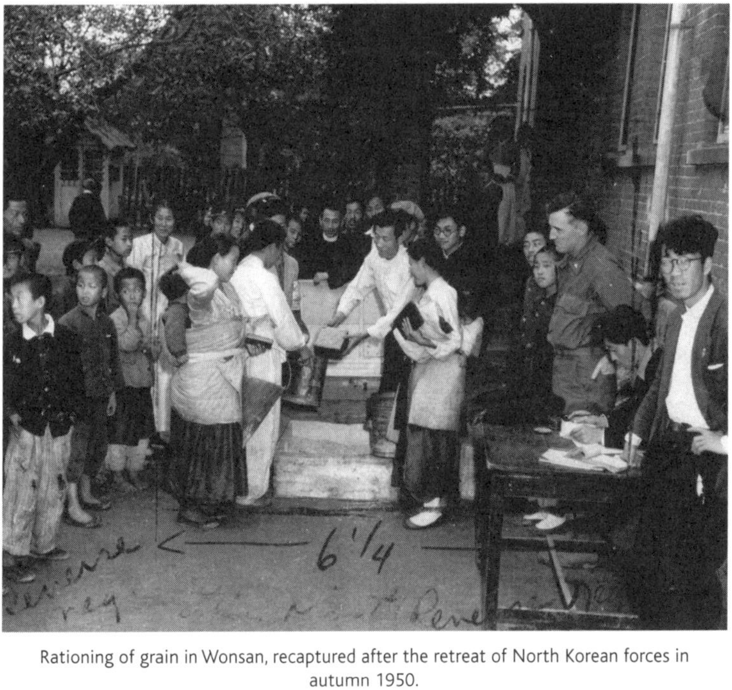

Rationing of grain in Wonsan, recaptured after the retreat of North Korean forces in autumn 1950.

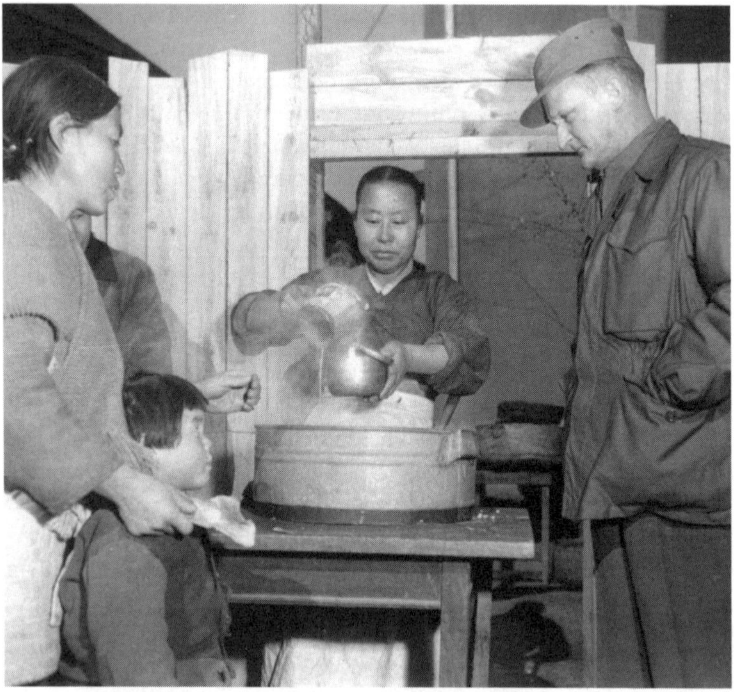

A feeding station in Seoul, December 1952.

to peasant uprisings that swept Kyŏngsang and Chŏlla provinces, followed by strikes and riots in several cities. American agricultural officials later remarked that the 'brutal methods' employed by police in the summer grain collections were among the 'basic factors' that played a role in the autumn unrest.[57]

The autumn harvest uprisings lasted only a few months, but led to inflation, unemployment and disastrous rises in living costs. By 1949 the retail price of beef in Seoul was 23 times what it had been in 1945, the price of cabbage 30 times, and the price of soybeans 40 times.[58] The government decontrolled most commodities except for those managed by government monopolies, which included tobacco, salt, opium, ginseng and sugar. While the retail price of salt remained relatively stable, more than one-third of the entire yearly supply of salt (often stolen from government salterns) was furnished to the population for exorbitant prices through black-market operations.[59] By 1947 the black-market economy that had emerged in the final years of the Sino-Japanese War was truly thriving (see p. 177, Table VI).

As a result of the economic chaos instigated by the free-market policy of the USAMGIK, the per capita average daily calorie intake in the southern half of the Korean peninsula fell from an estimated 2,039 calories during 1932–6 to 1,468 calories calculated for the period between May 1946 and April 1947. Unlike peasants and landowners, who could rely on their own agricultural produce to feed themselves, the urban population was highly dependent on the rationing system of the government, which was quickly resurrected after the failure of the open market introduced in October 1945. In February 1946 the Japanese staple food rationing system was reintroduced, with the daily ration set at 1 *hop* (approximately 145 grams) of rice or substitute grain per capita.[60] This amount was less than half the daily ration under Japanese rule, and provided roughly 500 calories, far from sufficient for survival.[61] In response to the serious social unrest that erupted in autumn 1946, the staple food ration was increased to 2.5 *hop* (approximately 355 grams) in December. A directive by Deputy Military Governor C. G. Helmick, distributed to all departments of the USAMGIK, the military governors of each province and the mayor of Seoul in February 1947, specified that for the period from 1 December 1946 to 31 July 1947 the 'general ration' was to be made up of 1.5 *hop* of rice and 1 *hop* of other grains. During the period from 1 August to 30 November 1947, before the new crop of rice became available, the share of rice would be reduced to 0.8 *hop*.[62]

In addition to the 'general ration', personnel of 'essential agencies and installations' such as policemen, lighthouse keepers and coast guards, as well as workers in 'priority industries' such as the mining and lumber industries, were entitled to 'special rations'. In the case of the latter, a bonus 'supplementary ration' of one more *hop* per person could be issued as a stimulant or a reward for production goals. Workers employed in transportation, communication and electrical utilities, as well as the machinery, chemical and textile industries, salterns and public works, were also eligible for 'supplementary rations'. 'Special rations' for hospital patients and orphaned children were specified at 3 *hop* (half of it rice), 70 grams more than the 'regular ration'. Prisoners were issued 4 *hop* of the 'least desirable and damaged, but edible, grains and canned foods', with a maximum of 1 *hop* of rice.[63]

As of May 1946, roughly one-third of the Koreans inhabiting the American occupation zone – approximately 7 million people – received the staple food ration.[64] The ration population reached its peak of roughly 9.5 million in 1948 (including partially self-supplying farmers who received supplementary rations), but dropped to 4.5 million in the autumn of 1949, and further to slightly over 1 million after the revision of the rationing programme in November 1949.[65] The food supply situation was at the time largely stabilized in terms of staple food, and improvements could be seen in the production of supplementary food as well. The livestock production programme resulted in an increase in the 'carry-over population' of pigs – that is, pigs that were not slaughtered – from 195,271 in 1946 to 379,882 in 1948. The 'carry-over population' of chickens also increased, from 1.6 to over 2 million. This dramatic increase by no means implies that meat and poultry consumption in South Korea was substantial. It was estimated that 15 million chickens were consumed annually, which translated to less than one chicken per capita per year. Nutritional surveys conducted by the Department of Public Health and Welfare confirmed that the daily diet of Koreans at the time was centred on rice and other grains, *kimch'i*, vegetables and beans, with eggs and meat playing a marginal role (see also chapter Five).[66]

The Japanese rationing system resurrected by the USAMGIK included the use of the *aegukpan* network.[67] 'Patriotic units' had not been dissolved after liberation and were occasionally utilized by the Americans for population surveys and other administrative functions. However, involvement in food rationing brought them back to the centre of community life. After the inauguration of the Republic of Korea, the system was further invigorated under the leadership of Citizens' Associations (Kungminhoe), and the units were renamed *kungminban* ('citizens' unit') in 1949. As was the case with *aegukpan*, membership in 'citizens' units' became compulsory for every South Korean citizen, and monthly meetings (*pansanghoe*) were conducted in a fashion strikingly resembling the *aegukpan* meetings.[68] During the Korean War the regular activities of 'citizens' units' were halted, but the network was utilized in the implementation of Daily Life Improvement (Saenghwal Kaesŏn Undong) campaigns that aimed at controlling the population in the midst of wartime turmoil and the loosening of social discipline. For example, on 18 November 1951 the government proclaimed a Wartime Daily Life Improvement Act (Chŏnsi Saenghwal Kaesŏn Pŏp) that imposed the spirit of austerity on the population.[69] By introducing measures such as prohibition of singing and dancing in restaurants, the sale of liquor before 5 p.m. and the importation, production and sale of luxuries, the government invested in turning 'wartime moderation' (*chŏnsi chŏlche*) into a national virtue. 'Citizens' units' were entrusted with the task of implementing the austerity policy, in a manner comparable with 'patriotic units'. The policy itself mimicked the Japanese wartime rhetoric of the previous decade, represented by the popular slogan 'Luxury is the enemy!' (*zeitaku wa teki da*).

By autumn 1952 the regular activities of *kungminban* were gradually resumed, ultimately turning the units into a control organ of the state. New regulations issued between 1953 and 1956 expanded their functions to include, along with food rationing, the dissemination of anti-communist propaganda and the implementation of government campaigns aimed at the rationalization of daily life.[70] Examples such as the transformation of *aegukpan* into *kungminban* provide hard evidence for institutional continuity in the management of the Korean population by the pre- and post-1945 regimes. They also underline the importance of food in the historical transformation of the Korean peninsula during the waging of war in the mid-twentieth century.

Along with reviving Japanese wartime policies, the American occupation also brought about new developments, introducing new foods into the dietary landscape of South Korea. In order to ease the gravity of shortages, large quantities of food were imported from U.S. sources in Burma, Siam, the Philippines, the Red Sea area and directly

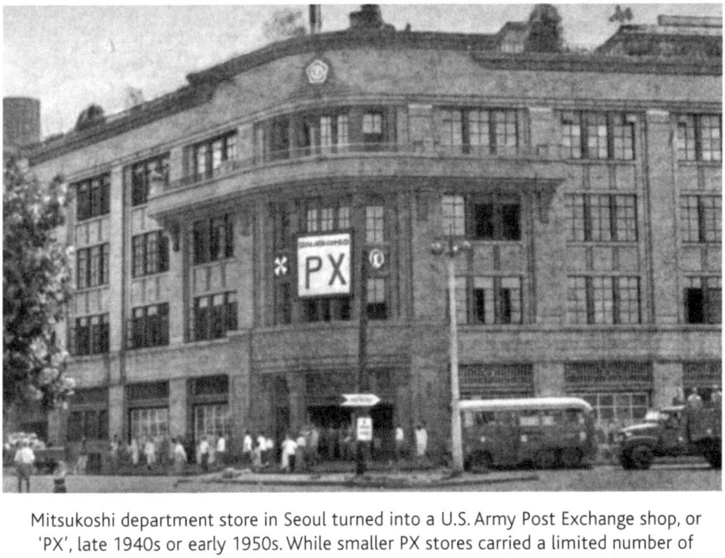

Mitsukoshi department store in Seoul turned into a U.S. Army Post Exchange shop, or 'PX', late 1940s or early 1950s. While smaller PX stores carried a limited number of items, such as razor blades, letter paper, soft drinks, cigarettes and candy, larger ones were comparable to department stores; they served as a morale booster for soldiers stationed overseas.

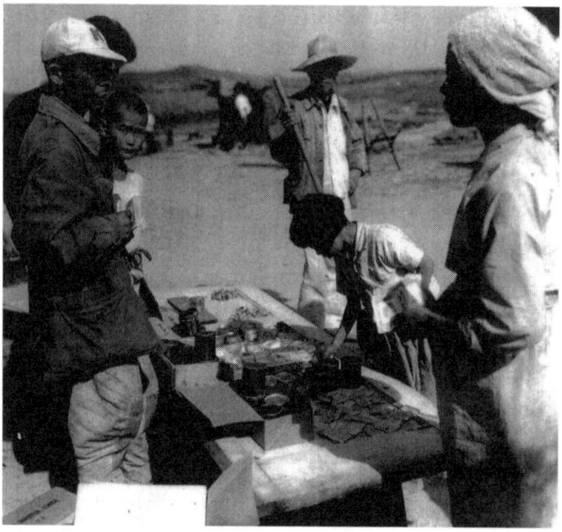

A black-market stall selling American goods, 1951.

from the U.S.[71] Between May and December 1946 a total of 179,132 tonnes of wheat and corn arrived in the American occupational zone. This was twice the volume of wheat, rye, barley and naked barley collected south of the 38th parallel during the entire 1946 summer grain harvest (87,428 tonnes).[72] Provisions from military stocks were also made available for consumption by Korean civilians. The official statistics list 155 tonnes of rice, 100 tonnes of beans, 411 tonnes of sugar and 10,370 tonnes of 'case goods' – canned foodstuffs that constituted the bulk of military rations. These figures do not include foodstuffs classified as 'deteriorated subsistence' unfit for army use, which were issued as supplementary food to dependent house servants and Korean citizens otherwise employed by the U.S. government.[73] Nor do they cover the candy bars and chewing gum generously handed out by GIs to Korean children or the military canned goods traded on the black market.[74] Like rice, which serves as a vivid reminder of Japanese colonial exploitation (see chapter One), in the collective memory such products function as powerful symbols of the Korean suffering inflicted by Cold War politics.

The Food Situation North of the 38th Parallel

By March 1951 the Korean War had made more than 3 million Koreans homeless. The first wave of refugees consisted of members of the South Korean population who were fleeing further south to escape the encroachment of the North Korean People's Army (NKPA) in the summer of 1950. Following the recapture of the 38th parallel by UN forces and their northward advance in October and November, the offensive launched by the Chinese Communist Forces (CCF) brought about the second wave of migration, this time of North Koreans. In the midst of harsh winter weather, thousands of North Koreans travelled south; the hardships of their journey were magnified by the great distances they had to travel and the restriction on their movements imposed by the policies of the Eighth United States Army in Korea (EUSAK). Refugees were not allowed to cross American battle lines and could only approach American positions accompanied by the police. All movement of Korean civilians had to end at sunset, with an informal understanding that 'lethal force could be used against Korean refugees as a last resort'.[75] Those who survived the journey were faced with further suffering, since Chinese intervention created a refugee crisis for the UN Command. As Sahr Conway-Lanz explains, 'awful conditions in refugee camps persisted beyond the early chaotic months of the war, and the U.S. military failed to cooperate with the International Committee of the Red Cross, which was attempting to ensure that treatment for the dislocated Koreans conformed to international law.'[76]

Ironically, North Korean refugees suffered hunger and poor dietary conditions only after they left their homes in the north. Before the outbreak of the Korean War the overall food supply situation of the North Korean population was much better than the conditions in the American occupation zone. This was despite the deplorable food situation in the northern half of the peninsula directly after Korea's liberation. In comparison to the southern half, the north is not blessed with geographical conditions suited for agriculture. Less than 20 per cent of North Korean territory can be cultivated and due to harsh weather conditions, growing seasons are short. In 1945, as was the case in the south and in other territories under Japanese control, the output of the North Korean harvest was below average, primarily due to lack of fertilizer and farm tools and the depleted wartime labour force, drained by growth in the industrial sector and military draft. A massive population movement to the south eased the pressure on North Korean food resources somewhat: nearly 250,000 Japanese soldiers and civilians moved southward to be repatriated, and large numbers of Koreans who had before 1945 been relocated to industrial complexes in the north crossed the 38th parallel and returned to their homes.[77]

Feeding the Red Army that now occupied the area was also a heavy burden. U.S. military intelligence estimated that the Soviet extraction of food in North Korea was approximately 10 per cent higher than the amount of food requisitioned by the Japanese during the Second World War; not infrequently food was sent by the occupying forces from Korea to the USSR.[78] While there is a possibility that these figures were not entirely unbiased, Soviet soldiers were infamous for their ruthless looting practices. As Catherine Merridale explains in her extensive study on the Red Army in the Second World War, while Soviet soldiers were not the only troops guilty of crimes, 'the Red Army did everything on a monumental scale'. On the Western front they went as far as shipping home a fleet of special trains carrying crates of champagne, fine china, bed linen, furs and even cars and dismantled factories.[79] In her novel *Who Ate Up All the Shinga?*, Park Wan-suh describes a word that symbolically marked the presence of Soviet soldiers in Seoul in the summer of 1950. The word derived from the Russian *dawai* (the imperative form of the verb 'to give'), and Park explains how 'people started bandying the term about, saying that a marketplace had been *dawaied*, that vegetable patches had been *dawaied*, even that women had been *dawaied*'.[80]

During the first months of the occupation the Soviet forces in Korea acquired provisions through their tried-and-tested methods of looting, pillage, requisition of food supplies and slaughter of livestock. After the North Korean Provisional People's Committee (NKPPC) – the basis of the central government in Pyongyang – came to power in February 1946, food extraction for the Red Army became more systematized. At first a 'responsibility system' was put in place, in which each village held meetings to plan the upcoming farm production under the direction of each county's 'people's committee'. These were recognized by the Soviets and came under increasing communist influence. Following the land reform a month later, farmers were effectively taxed at approximately 50 per cent of their crop, with 15 per cent of this amount reserved for the Soviets.[81]

The motto of the reform was the 'land to the tillers' principle that aimed to abolish the phenomenon of tenancy altogether. According to the ordinance passed on 5 March 1946, the following categories of land were subject to confiscation: 1) land possessed by the government, civilians, and organizations of Japan; 2) land owned by national traitors, that is, those who collaborated with the Japanese colonialists; 3) land owned by those who fled after the liberation; 4) land owned by Korean landlords in excess of five *chŏngbo* (around 5 hectares) per farming household; 5) land owned by absentee landlords; 6) land rented out continuously for many years, regardless of size; and 7) land owned by churches, monasteries and other religious organizations in excess of five *chŏngbo*.[82]

The confiscated land was redistributed to over 700,000 small-holding and tenant farmers who acquired the 'permanent right' to farm the land (and could pass this right to their offspring), but the land could not be rented, sold or mortgaged. In total the operation involved nearly 1 million *chŏngbo* of land, with each household receiving an average of 1.33 *chŏngbo*. Unlike former landlords, former middle-class peasants who owned more than five *chŏngbo* of arable land but tilled it themselves were allowed to keep it, but the North Korean Constitution promulgated in September 1948 restricted the size of landholdings to five *chŏngbo* in the plains or twenty *chŏngbo* in the mountainous regions.[83]

In theory, farmers were required to hand over 25 per cent of their crops to the authorities in exchange for the right to farm the land. This system of 'agricultural tax-in-kind' (*nongŏp hyŏnmulse*), introduced on 27 June 1946, replaced all previous taxes in the countryside. In practice, the tax turned out far higher than the nominal average of 25 per cent – at times exceeding 50 per cent – due to the notorious tendency of central and local planning authorities to overestimate the anticipated production in the next harvest.[84] Nonetheless, 'private' ownership of the land encouraged greater productivity. According to North Korean sources, the harvest in 1948 exceeded the peak output of the colonial period. While U.S. analysts estimated it to be just under the wartime average yield of 3.1 million tonnes,[85] it could not be denied that the new regime in Pyongyang had succeeded in feeding its population, an achievement that could not be claimed by the authorities in Seoul.

In his study of the early years of the North Korean regime, Charles Armstrong – a leading expert on the early history of North Korea – argues that the land reform of 1946 was one of the 'most rapid, and thoroughgoing land redistribution efforts in history', and that it 'effected a revolutionary change in the social and economic life of rural Korea'.[86] As Armstrong points out, despite its thoroughness, the North Korean land reform was an absolutely non-violent one. Nothing remotely approaching the bloodshed that accompanied land reforms in the Soviet Union, China and Vietnam ever took place in North Korea, most probably due to the fact that the majority of stakeholders had already left by 1946, either being repatriated to Japan or migrating to the south.[87]

The success story of the North Korean land reform is in striking contrast with the developments related to land reform in the South. Sales of the first plots of land formerly owned by Japanese landlords to the Korean tenants began in April 1948, two years after the North Korean tenants had acquired their land. This delay was mainly due to the inability of the Interim Legislative Assembly in the American Occupation Zone to come to an agreement on the matter.[88] In spring 1948 the U.S. Military Government set up a special agency in order to handle the sale. All the landholdings of the New Korea Company (which in November 1945 took over all former Japanese property) were transferred to the newly formed National Land Administration (NLA) and offered for sale to Korean farmers. The NLA provided each farmer with a fifteen-year loan to pay for the land. In the face of rampant inflation, the price of each plot was expressed in measures of grain, set at three times its average annual yield, and the mortgage was also to be paid in grain. This programme affected only one aspect of the land-ownership problem in South Korea, since the Japanese owned no more than 15.3 per cent of the farmland. Ideological disputes within the newly formed Republic of Korea delayed the promulgation of the Land Reform Act that applied to the remaining share of landlord-held land to 15 June 1949. Moreover, its implementation was halted by a combination of bureaucratic problems and political pressure by the landlord class to delay the reform. Not a single acre changed hands before the outbreak of the Korean War.[89]

On the whole, largely due to the land reform, the standard of living of poor peasantry in the North considerably improved, not only in comparison to the colonial period but also to the conditions in the South.[90] In addition, a critical consequence of the reform was that it facilitated popular support for the new government. Even American analysts emphasized the political gains that the reform brought about, admitting that 'half the population of north Korea was given a tangible stake in the regime and at the same time the north Korean government gained an important propaganda weapon in its campaign against the south'.[91]

Along with the land reform, a swift reintroduction of the food rationing that had functioned under Japanese rule during the Pacific

War was another important step that ensured popular support for the regime and prevented social unrest. In October 1945, when the U.S. Military Government in the South declared a free market in rice, the authorities in the North prohibited private trade in grain in urban areas and procured all the grain in circulation. This drastic measure made it possible to distribute rations of 500 grams of grain per day.[92] The North Korean food rationing system utilized the local branches of the colonial-era Korea Food Corporation, which had been taken over by People's Committees immediately after Japan's capitulation.[93]

In February 1946 new national norms of food rations were specified that basically classified members of the population into one of four categories (see p. 178, Table VII). In the summer of 1946, along with the introduction of 'tax-in-kind', a North Korean food distribution system began to take shape as a tool of social control. Food rationing was then not only officially transformed from an emergency measure into a permanent institution, but restrictions were made on the basis of 'social status and political reliability' as to who was entitled to receive rations.[94] The newly established Food Administration Bureau (Yangjŏngbu) guaranteed food rations only to the urbanites employed at legally permitted workplaces, and bureaucrats and officials working for the state. Those employed in the non-socialist sector were entitled to rations only if they were contracted by the government.[95] The number of people dependent for their food supply on the distribution system of the state grew rapidly after August 1946, when the nationalization of major industries was stipulated and an increasing share of the North Korean population became employees of the state.

The 'official' peacetime daily ration of a North Korean People's Army soldier consisted of 1 kg of rice, 400 grams of vegetables, 150 grams of fish and 150 grams of condiments (soy sauce, bean curd, salt, oils and so on). Most food supplies were obtained locally from the People's Committee of each area by means of 'spot taxes' or payment in the form of 'procurement notes' issued by the responsible food supply officer of each unit.[96] However, once the NKPA forces crossed the 38th parallel, the procedure had to be altered. The strategy was to make maximum use of supplies captured from the enemy. As was the case with Imperial Japanese Army soldiers fighting throughout the Pacific a decade earlier, communist troops in the Korean War not infrequently had to rely on foraging to supplement their meagre rations. Soldiers were often encouraged to attack in expectation of capturing food, clothing and medical supplies as well as arms and ammunition.[97]

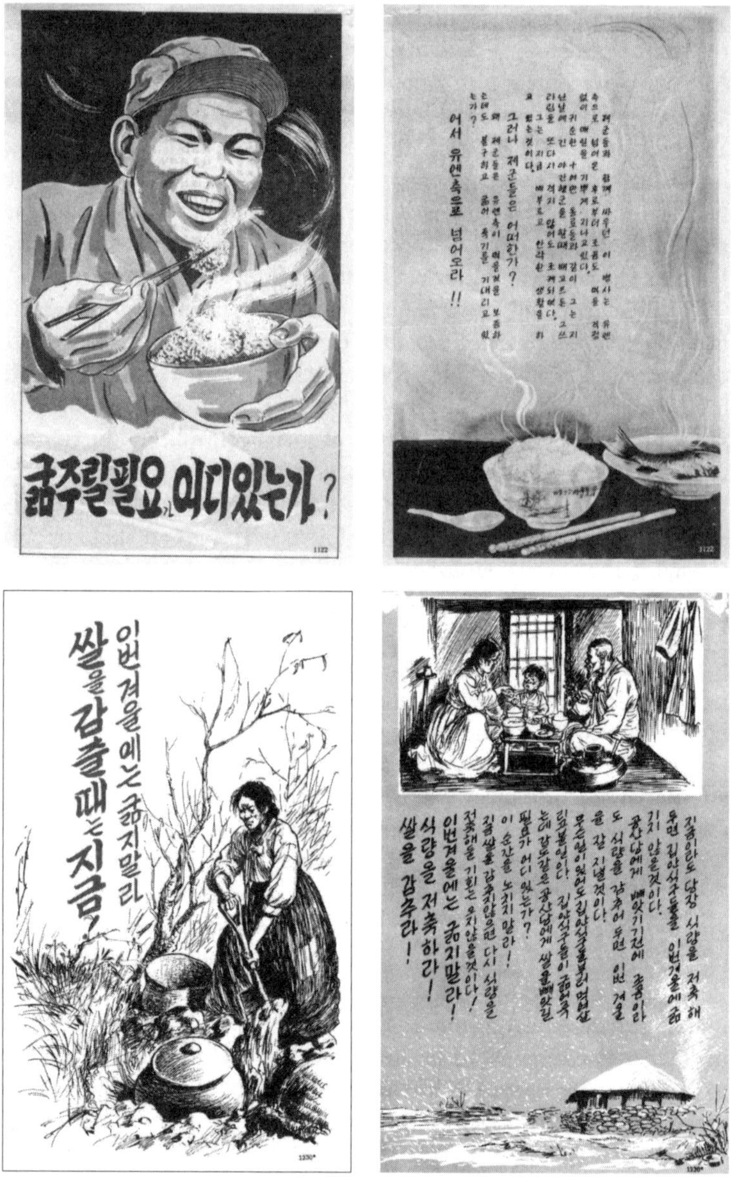

U.S. intelligence pamphlets dropped over North Korean forces in 1951 and 1952.

Intelligence agencies of the United Nations Command estimated that after hostilities began, the NKPA soldiers' 'official rations' were no longer available, and North Korean soldiers subsisted mainly on baked rice or millet and rice flour or rice biscuits.[98] Accordingly, food played an important role in the psychological warfare programmes of the Far East Command (FEC) and the Eighth United States Army in Korea (EUSAK), designed to destroy the combat effectiveness of the enemy. Food constituted a major theme in both anti-morale and surrender appeal tactics.[99] For example, a leaflet addressed to the North Korean soldier, issued in October 1951, featured a man enjoying a bowl of rice with a question 'Why Go Hungry?' written underneath (see opposite, top left and right). The text on the reverse side of the pamphlet read:

> This Korean communist soldier, now safe behind the UN lines, enjoys hot rice with side dishes, each day. Along with thousands of his comrades he no longer suffers hunger during the long night marches he once had to make. With his stomach filled with hot rice and vegetables he now enjoys life away from the war. But what about you, soldier? Why go hungry this fall when the UN offers you an abundance of good food? SAVE YOUR LIFE – ESCAPE TO THE UN LINES.[100]

Two other pamphlets issued a year later were both addressed to the civilian population, with the messages: 'Don't Starve This Winter! Hoard Your Food Now!' (opposite, bottom left and right) and 'Hide Your Rice! Don't Starve for Communists!'[101] The former urged North Korean civilians to hoard food in order to assure their survival during the winter months, and the latter advised farmers on how to hide their rice from communist collectors. Such leaflets would be dropped at the targeted areas either in leaflet bombs – each containing 20–40,000 leaflets – or in artillery shells, which proved much more accurate in reaching their destination. Between June 1950 and July 1953 the U.S. army distributed approximately 100 million leaflets using the latter method.[102]

It is difficult to assess whether the promise of 'hot rice with side dishes' for North Korean soldiers who surrendered was always fulfilled. Official records indicate that prisoners of war were supplied daily, following the Geneva Convention, with '1.08 pounds of grain, .2 pounds of dried peas or beans, .1 pound of fish or meat, .5 pounds of vegetables, and .03 pounds of salt'.[103] Unlike the supplies for the UN troops, which were shipped primarily from the United States (see below), food and cigarettes for the consumption of the Republic of Korea Army and the prisoners of war were obtained from local markets in Japan. A total of 182,000 kg of cuttlefish and 3,256,000 packages of Japanese cigarettes are reported to have been shipped to Korea by the Tokyo Quartermaster Depot in March 1951.[104] The rations for North Korean POWs seem to have improved over the years, at least on paper. Records from 1953 mention a daily allowance of '1.4 pounds of grain (of which at least 50 per cent is rice), .1 pound of dried fish, .6 pound of fresh vegetable obtained from Korean sources, .2 pound of dried peas or beans, and condiments'.[105]

Feeding the Southern Troops

> At about noon, the truck pulled off the road at the camp of a United States Army battalion. The driver mentioned an invitation that I join him for a meal . . . I tagged along close to my host as we got into the self-service cafeteria-style serving line. Following the driver's lead, I cut myself a thick slab of meat loaf, spooned out steamed mixed vegetables and fresh salad, and took a big bowl of vegetable soup with bread-and-butter. I was surprised to see that there was still room on my tray, so I grabbed a huge piece of chocolate cake and topped the whole thing off with a cup of hot coffee with lots of cream and sugar. I had not seen so much good food since my last dinner with my family before we left Harbin in 1945. Without uttering a single word, I shovelled all this delicious repast into my mouth, using my spoon and fork and, where necessary, my fingers. I ate every last crumb and drank every last drop, and even felt a little distress as I pushed my tray away.
>
> As we left the mess hall after a satisfying smoke, the chubby mess attendant pressed several chocolate bars into my hand. I could not understand what he said to me, but I suppose it must have been something like, 'Hey, Shorty, you look so hungry, and you ate so much, you deserve to have these to eat along the way.'[106]

Since the late 1930s Korea had functioned as a logistical base for the Imperial Japanese Army and Navy, and its economy was intertwined with the total war machine of the Japanese Empire. In 1950 the situation was reversed: it was Japan that now functioned as a logistical base for the American and South Korean forces and UN battalions that fought on the Korean peninsula. Japan Logistical Command in Tokyo functioned as the headquarters of most of the logistical operations during the Korean War, including the provisioning of troops. The Americans handled the lion's share of logistical support for all the units under its command: the U.S. Eighth Army, the UN battalions, the Republic of Korea (ROK) forces and the so-called Korean Augmentation to the U.S. Army (KATUSA), Korean civilians drafted as support stuff for military units. In June 1952 the troop strength of UN Command in Korea stood at 695,715 men.[107]

As an exception to the general principle of the U.S. Quartermaster Corps being responsible for logistical support of all troops under its command, the Republic of Korea Army (ROKA) handled the subsistence supply of its soldiers on its own.[108] This was a legacy of the Imperial Japanese Army (IJA), much of whose organizational structure ROK forces inherited.[109] Approximately 187,000 Korean soldiers served in the IJA during the Pacific War, and the bulk of ROK officers and managerial cadre were IJA veterans, including the first Quartermaster General of the South Korean Army, Lt Col. Paik Sun Jin, and his follower, Yun Soo Hyun.[110] The IJA's basic principle of subsistence supply was the local procurement of food, which entailed the quartermaster of each unit being responsible for securing food for his men.[111] Under American influence channelled through the Korean Military Advisory Group (KMAG), activated in July 1949, the ROKA established a central procurement agency for rice, but throughout the Korean War each company commander was granted a monetary allowance per man to purchase food locally. It was only in the summer of 1953 – after the armistice was already in place – that centralized procurement, inspection, storage and distribution of perishable subsistence for South Korean troops were officially sanctioned, and South Korean troops were finally serviced in a manner comparable to the U.S. model.[112]

The principle of local procurement constituted a major problem in the subsistence supply of the ROKA. First of all, the monetary allowance per man never seemed to keep up with inflation in the Korean won, and it was almost impossible for a commander to obtain all the necessary supplementary food to accompany the staple ration.[113] Moreover, as Donald Chung reveals in his memoirs,

> corruption was rampant throughout the ROK Army; supplies of every type were routinely siphoned off at every command level leading down to the companies and platoons manning the front, and only a tiny fraction of our allocations actually reached us. Most mornings, each of us received as our daily ration less than a cupful of rice, which we had to cook in our canteen cups, and some pickled vegetables.[114]

The subsistence supply of the U.S. armed forces and UN battalions stands in strong contrast to this meagre fare. The foundation of the subsistence supply for the troops during the Korean War was the 'basic operational B ration', largely comprised of canned and dehydrated food. However, in comparison to the situation during the Pacific War, the U.S. Army Quartermaster Corps in Korea introduced fresh subsistence on a previously unheard-of scale. Perishable meats, poultry and fish were served 50.5 times a month for dinner and supper meals, and fresh eggs were served at 21 breakfasts per month. Instead of supplying units with bread for three meals of the day, bread ingredients for the third meal were distributed instead, making it possible for units to add variety to their rations by baking hot rolls, biscuits and extra pastries.[115]

Fresh bananas were first supplied on a test basis in 1951. After an enthusiastic reception, it was decided to provide them twice monthly to all the troops during the warm-weather months. The bananas, grown in Taiwan, were shipped green to Japan by water transport, conditioned and ripened by Japanese processors, and then airlifted to airfields in Korea adjacent to Class I issue points for rapid distribution at a ready-to-eat stage of ripeness. Apples and tangerines, as well as fresh fish and eggs, were purchased regularly, either in Korea or in Japan.[116]

The degree of fresh subsistence described above would not have been possible without the technological advancements achieved since the end of the Pacific War. The Korean War was the first armed conflict in which modern refrigeration and transportation facilities were used to the maximum possible extent. By the summer of 1952 every soldier in Korea was allowed approximately 0.08 cubic metres of 'reefer' space for his food supplies per month.[117] 'Swift refrigerator ships', reported *The Quartermaster Review* in spring 1953,

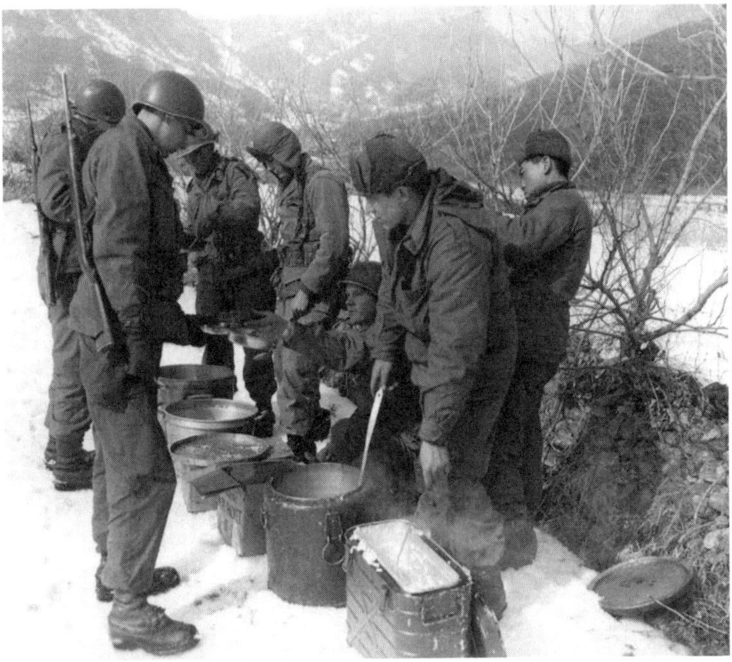

A hot meal is delivered to the front line by the Quartermaster Corps of the U.S. Army, February 1951.

> carry the perishables from the U.S. to Korea at a rate of one vessel every ten days. In Korea, extensive use is made of portable 'walk-in' refrigerator boxes which are banked at strategic locations in the base depot and supply points. These are supplemented by the use of commercial ice plants and by the use of refrigerator barges for offshore storage and coastal transport. Refrigerator cars provide daily transport along the main rail lines.[118]

The Korean War was also the first instance of aerial supply being used by U.S. armed forces as a standard component of logistical support. The first Aerial Supply Company was activated on 31 July 1950 and a few weeks later completed its first mission: the dropping of psychological warfare leaflets over enemy forces. By spring 1951, alongside equipment and other supplies, the Airborne Quartermasters were delivering in Korea over 7 tonnes of onions, lettuces and radishes daily from hydroponic farms in Japan. By October, average daily deliveries had increased more than fourfold, and included tomatoes, cucumbers and aubergines.[119]

The proximity of Japan, with abundant labour and food resources, was the second vital condition that made possible the large-scale supply of fresh food to the troops in Korea. Along with fresh eggs, bananas and vegetables for American troops, Japan was also the chief supplier of the combat ration for South Korean soldiers. Approximately 1 million of such rations per month were assembled by the employees of the Tokyo Quartermaster Depot and shipped to Korea.[120] The combat ration was an exception to the rule of ROKA organizing their own subsistence supply independent of the U.S. channels: it was to be provided for ROKA soldiers by U.S. quartermasters along with other equipment considered crucial for combat operations.

An individual pre-cooked ration generally known as the C-Ration was intended to be consumed by frontline troops when fresh food (A-Ration) or packaged unprepared food (B-Ration) was not available, usually due to the circumstances of combat preventing the unit from

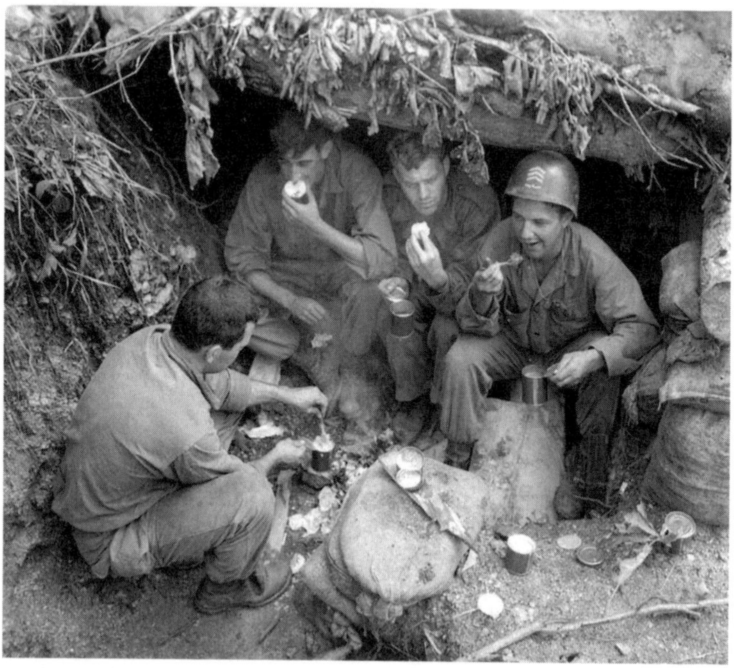

U.S. soldiers eating C-Rations at the front line of the Korean War, north of Hwach'ŏn Dam, 17 August 1951.

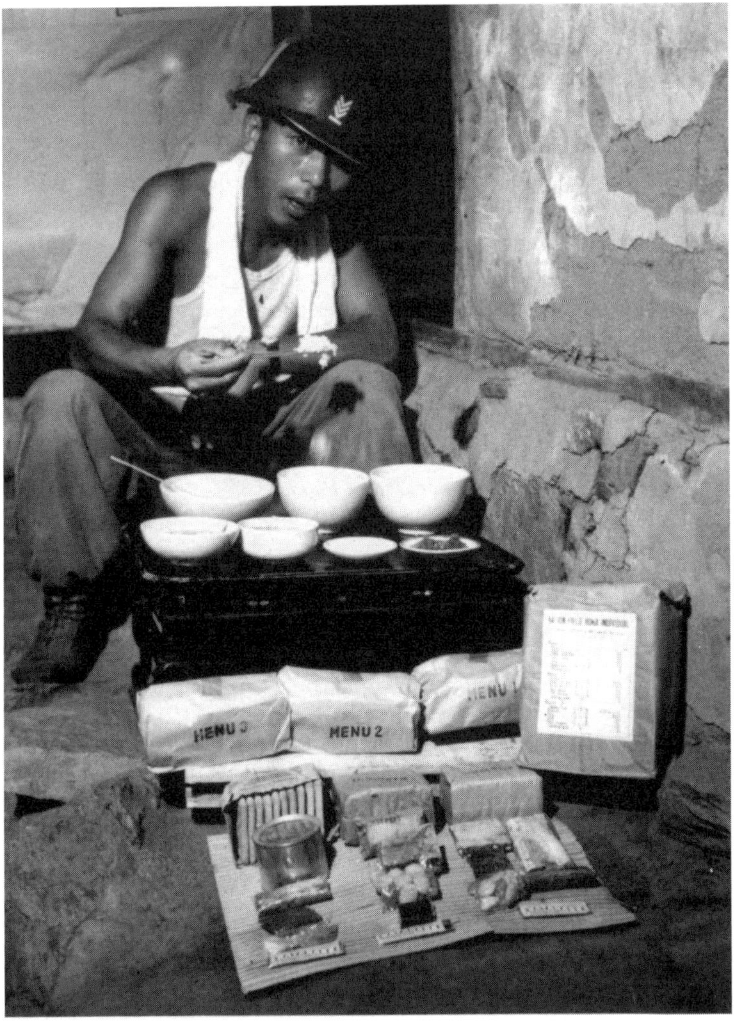

A soldier of the Republic of Korea Army eating lunch in the ruins of a house, 1951. Field rations made in Japan for the ROK Army are shown unpacked in front of him.

being able to cook. The C-Ration's major component – along with canned fruit, chocolate, instant coffee, crackers, jam and chewing gum – was a can containing a ready-to-eat meal: beans and frankfurters, beans with pork, meat and beans, ham and lima beans, spaghetti and meat, hamburgers with gravy, pork sausage patties with gravy, meat and noodles, chicken with vegetables, beef stew or corned beef hash.[121] At first, standard C-Rations were provided to the ROKA soldiers. However, they soon proved unsuited to the taste preferences and dietary habits of Koreans and were replaced in November 1950, during the drive for the Yalu River in North Korea, by ROKA Ration, 12-in-1, which was specially designed for the ROKA soldiers. The first shipment travelled by airlift from Kimpo Airfield to Pyongyang and then further by truck.

> The new combat ration is packed in wooden boxes, twelve rations to the box, with each ration packed individually in a water-resistant paper bag. The breakfast, dinner, and supper meals are packed in separate paper bags within the one water-resistant bag. The components of the ration are as follows:

Biscuits	600 grams
*Canned mackerel, mackerel-pike, sardines, herring, sukesotara or Alaska Pollack**	210 grams
or *canned tuna flakes*	200 grams
Prunes, dried	30 grams
Roast soy beans	30 grams
Roast peas	40 grams
Hard candy	60 grams
Kelp	60 grams
Salt	10 grams
Red pepper [chilli]	10 grams
Green tea	8 grams
Chewing gum	15 grams

*Each ration contains two cans of two different kinds of fish.[122]

The ROKA combat ration is an interesting example of the pervasive legacy of recycling, for use in the Korean War, of practices and channels of military subsistence that were developed for the purpose of the Sino-Japanese War. The ration was designed by Kawashima Shirō (1895–1986), an ex-general of the Imperial Japanese Army, a leading member of the Army Provisions Depot in Tokyo and a supervising researcher of the airborne rations division of the Imperial Japanese Navy.[123] The ROKA ration was manufactured in Japan; the food was obtained from local markets in Japan by the newly established organizational unit of the Tokyo Quartermaster Depot – the Purchasing Division (which was charged with the supervision of procurement from Japanese sources) – and packaged, under Storage Division supervision, with an assembly-line technique, by Japanese employees.[124] The know-how and experience acquired by the Japanese during the Pacific War in manufacturing processed food for the Imperial Japanese Army and Navy proved a valuable asset for the ROKA.

5
South Korea: From Food Aid to the Revival of Royal Cuisine

> Kijun watched closely to see where something he might like to pick up later landed. 'I hope we find some meat again today,' he said. 'Do you boys remember what I found in a can last time? My uncle said it was "ham." It really tasted good when my mother made a piggie stew with it.'
>
> 'What's piggie stew?' Chandol asked.
>
> 'You collect everything you can eat from the bengko garbage – meat and cheese and chicken bones and everything – and boil them together in a pot. That's piggie stew,' Jun explained. 'Some people call it U.N. soup. My uncle saw the town folks sell it on the streets the other day. He told my mother the piggie stew recipe.'[1]

From Food Aid to *Ramyŏn*

The 'piggie stew' from Ahn Junghyo's novel *Silver Stallion* is nowadays commonly known under the name *pudae tchigae* (literally 'battalion stew'), officially translated by *The Korean Food Guide in English* as 'GI stew' – 'a spicy stew of wieners, luncheon meat, macaroni and vegetables. This dish originated from ingredients that could be scavenged from the U.S. military camps in Korea during the Korean War.'[2] Since the late 1990s *pudae tchigae* has experienced a renaissance as a nostalgia food. It is served at trendy restaurants in hip locations to the young generation of South Koreans to whom the idea of food shortage is entirely unfamiliar.

Pudae tchigae was in the first place a staple of military camptowns (*kijich'on*), which for decades constituted a fixture of the South

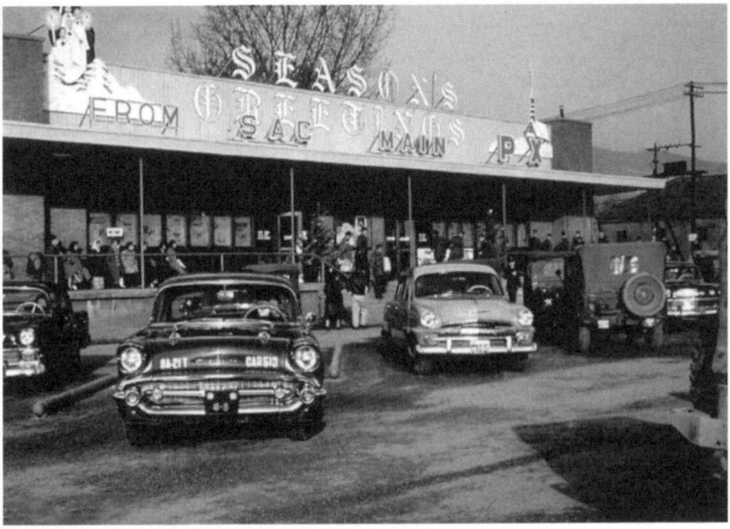

A U.S. Army Post Exchange store (PX) around Christmas time, 1958.

Korean landscape. The town of Pup'yŏng, near Inch'ŏn, which emerged near U.S. military installations soon after the arrival of American forces on Korean soil in 1945, went into history as the very first *kijich'on*. Their number rapidly increased during the Korean War, when over 300,000 U.S. soldiers were stationed on the peninsula.[3] Some of the earliest and largest camptowns included It'aewŏn in the heart of Seoul and sections of Pusan nicknamed Hialeah and Texas. During the 1960s, the heyday of military camptowns, 62,000 U.S. soldiers were stationed in virtually every corner of South Korea, and in particular concentration in the proximity of the Demilitarized Zone (DMZ), a strip of land approximately 4 km wide traversing the peninsula on both sides of the 38th parallel. The town of Tongduch'ŏn in the Paju area northeast of Seoul is the home of the largest *kijich'on*, with the appropriate name of 'Little Chicago'.[4]

The association of military camptowns with prostitution, social deviance and immorality situated them at the margins of Korean society. They were perceived as a 'necessary evil', the price Korea had to pay for the military security provided for the nation by the United States. However, the U.S. military bases not only provided employment for those directly involved in the sex industry, but served as an important source of income and food for a larger section of the population. Often in complicity with GIs, Korean civilians smuggled supplies out of the bases,

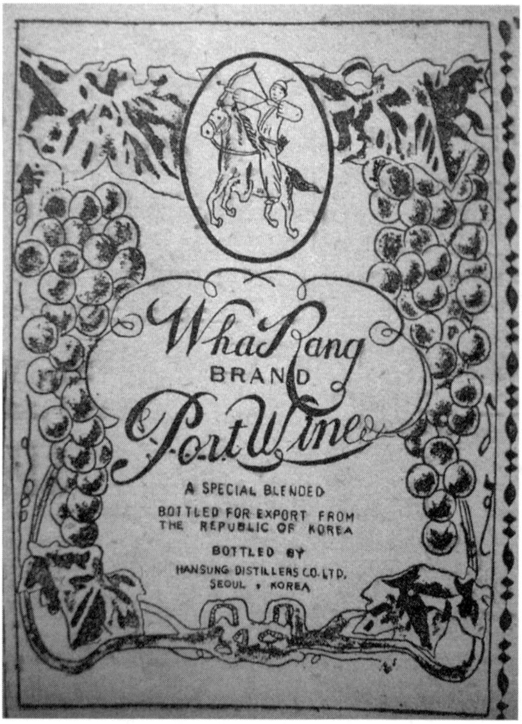

An advertisement for a Korean brand of port wine in *The Korean Republic*, 9 September 1953.

selling them for a handsome profit on the black market. Inhabitants of nearby villages opened laundries, restaurants and other businesses catering to the everyday needs of the soldiers and the camptown women.[5] Not infrequently, American GIs were also primary customers of Koreans engaged in more respectable occupations, such as the protagonists of Pak Wan-so's celebrated novel *Naked Tree*, who work in a studio that produces hack portrait paintings.[6] Many Korean distilleries and breweries were kept in business owing to military bulk orders and private purchases by American soldiers, as civilian consumption largely stagnated due to the ailing economy. An edition of the English-language newspaper *The Korean Republic* from September 1953 carried advertisements for Korean gin, port and whisky by Kumkang Brewing and Hansung Distilleries.[7] Korean beer produced by Oriental Brewery and Chosun Brewery, originally subsidiaries of the Japanese brewers set up in the colony during the 1930s (see chapter One), was from 1958 onwards contracted by the U.S. armed forces to replace the Japanese beer that had been provided to the troops thus far. In the early 1960s orders for the U.S. forces made up 23 per cent of the entire production of the two breweries.[8]

In contrast to the relatively affluent, well-fed American soldiers, the majority of South Koreans remained concerned with staving off hunger and making ends meet. Throughout the 1950s South Korea remained heavily dependent upon foreign aid, and even in the early 1960s the country was ranked among the world's poorest nations along with Burma, Congo, India and Kenya.[9] This was partly due to the property damage caused by the Korean War, which has been estimated at a total of over U.S.$3 billion. The shattered industrial base was further devastated by the economic policies of the corrupt administration of South Korea's first president, Syngman Rhee (1875–1965). An assessment of the situation offered in 1955 by U.S. officials bluntly stated that

> inadequate fiscal and credit policies – combined with unwise and politically motivated controls on foreign trade, domestic business and foreign investment have produced disastrous inflation, stifled initiative, disrupted normal price relationships, prevented capital formation and so paralyzed the productive process in general that massive U.S. aid is producing little net progress in the economy.[10]

Besides being a reminder of the poverty-stricken 1950s, *pudae tchigae* also reveals the legacy of the militarized reality of South Korean life during the decades of Cold War tension. Seungsook Moon has coined the term 'militarized modernity' to pinpoint the essence of the period of General Park Chung-hee's military dictatorship.[11] Park's administration, which ruled in South Korea between 1961 and 1979 and was characterized by strong state intervention in the economy and in the daily life of its citizens, not only formed the foundation for the Korean economic 'miracle' but has moulded generations of South Koreans into disciplined 'dutiful nationals' (*kungmin*). As we have observed in chapter Four, this process is part of the colonial legacy intensified at the time of the Korean War. Moon argues that the militarization of the nation and the labour market – implemented through the institution of universal male conscription – was a key factor in South Korean economic growth which would not have been possible outside of the context of the Cold War.[12] Between 1965 and 1985 South Korea's gross national product increased at an annualized average of over 8 per cent, and by the 1990s South Korean incomes reached parity with those of many European countries.[13]

It is often emphasized that the phenomenal growth of the South Korean economy since the late 1960s depended largely on the industrialization strategies of the Park regime, which shifted resources from production for domestic consumption to production for export, sacrificing present for future consumption.[14] However, another factor – which is less eagerly revealed – played a critical role in South Korea's rise to affluence. The economic profit from the Vietnam War (1955–75) is a covert cause of the South Korean economic 'miracle'. A total of 350,000 ROK soldiers were deployed in Vietnam between 1965 and 1975, generating a spectacular financial revenue for the economy. The benefit took various forms, from direct payments – such as a per capita remittance for each soldier sent, soldiers' pay and preferential treatment of Korean producers when securing orders for U.S. forces in Vietnam – to long-term economic gains, such as direct and indirect U.S. financial aid, advantageous loans and favourable conditions for Korean export goods on the U.S. market.[15]

The phenomenal contribution of the Vietnam War to the South Korean economy not only reveals the intricate connections between the rising standard of living in South Korea and Cold War politics, but unites the two pillars in Park's vision for the development of South Korea: a strong military and a state-guided economy, heavily influenced by the strategies of the Japanese wartime empire. It was largely through men like Park Chung-hee (1917–1979), a graduate of the Japanese Military Academies and a veteran of the Imperial Japanese Army, that the legacy of colonial rule was kept alive in South Korea. His background accounts for the great degree of continuity between the Japanese measures of mobilization and surveillance employed during the late 1930s and '40s and the strategies brought into play for the same purposes twenty years later.[16] For example, his policies of heavier state intervention in the agricultural sector relied on channels and methods dating back to the agro-bureaucracy of the colonial era. Agricultural policies instigated through state intervention aimed at food autarky, a goal that guided the policies of the Japanese Empire (see chapter One) as well as the agricultural reforms in the Democratic People's Republic of Korea (see chapter Six). As Larry Burmeister explains,

> the 1970s was a decade of explicit import substitution in agriculture, as protectionist policies combined with new technology development and diffusion were promulgated to effect rice self-sufficiency. A major object of the rice

> self-sufficiency drive was to save foreign exchange expenditures that would have been necessary for staple food imports if significant production increases in rice production had not occurred. Foreign exchange savings were channelled into high-priority industrial investments.[17]

These policies went hand in hand with strict state regulation of rice consumption. Restaurants were prohibited from serving rice-based dishes entirely on Wednesdays and Thursdays and between 11 a.m. and 5 p.m. on the remaining days. Moreover, rice could only be served mixed with barley in the proportion 3:1. Schools also introduced regulations concerning students' lunches, which were to contain a rice–barley mixture in the ratio 7:3.[18] Similar rice-saving measures had been introduced during the Korean War and were again confirmed by government instructions in 1957. The industrial use of rice, for example in brewing alcohol or manufacturing rice-based confectionery, had been prohibited since the early 1950s.[19]

Along with restrictions that aimed to reduce the demand for rice, the government also actively promoted the consumption of flour-based

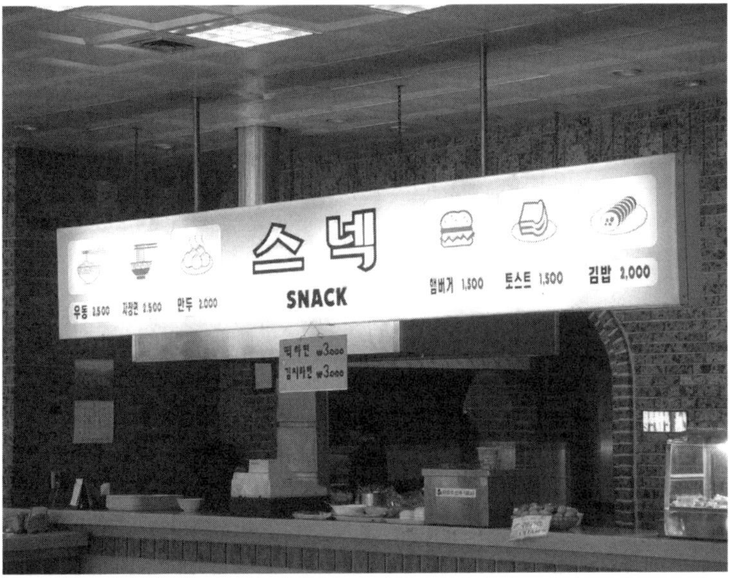

Snack shop at a highway rest area in 2006, featuring the mainstays of the *punsikchŏm*-era menus: Japanese-style noodles (*udong*), Chinese-style noodles (*chajangmyŏn*) and dumplings (*mandu*).

dishes. Subsidized cafeterias that specialized in serving bread, noodles, and dumplings, appropriately named *punsik sent'ŏ* ('flour food centre') and *punsikchŏm* ('flour food store'), were set up throughout the country. The first such cafeteria, Misŏngtang, began to operate in the city of Taegu in 1961. A second was opened at another location in the city in 1963 and the two were tremendously popular.[20] Such cafeterias provided a rare opportunity for ordinary Koreans to eat out, a practice that was not widespread even in cities. In 1977 eating out accounted for less than 3 per cent of the food expenditure of urban households, and a decade later was still no more than 8.9 per cent.[21] A phenomenal growth in eating out expenditure would take off after the late 1980s, skyrocketing to 20.3 per cent in 1990, 31.5 per cent in 1995, 39.4 per cent in 2000 and 47 per cent by 2007.[22]

In order to increase the consumption of wheat, the government also stimulated the industrial processing of flour into ready-to-eat snacks. The Ministry of Agriculture stipulated that at least one industrial bakery and one *ramyŏn* factory should be established in each province.[23] *Ramyŏn* is the Korean name for instant noodle soup, which now has a firm place in the pantheon of South Korean cuisine, having achieved the status of a national dish in less than three decades. The manufacture of *ramyŏn* in Korea was begun in September 1963 by Samyang Foods (Samyang sikp'um). With a strong backing from the flour-promotion campaign of the government, in four years the sales of Samyang *ramyŏn* increased by 30 times, soaring from 324 million won in 1966 to 9.792 billion won in 1970.[24] The total production of instant noodles in South Korea expanded from 2.4 million portions in 1966 to 3.78 billion in 1990, translating into 83 portions per capita per year.[25] Today over 100 brands compete on the South Korean *ramyŏn* market, with Nongshim (which has more than half of the market share and produces the best-selling spicy Shin Ramyŏn), Ottugi and Samyang the leading players.[26]

In 2010 South Korea ranked as the world's sixth largest consumer of instant noodles, with 3.41 billion portions consumed that year.[27] In terms of per capita consumption, however, South Koreans have for years ranked as number one, in 2010 consuming nearly 70 portions per person, approximately one portion every 5.2 days. These statistics have been confirmed by consumer polls. A survey conducted in 2000 in Seoul among 589 men and women between the ages of 10 and 50 revealed that the majority of respondents (57.9 per cent) ate *ramyŏn* at least once a week, while 29.8 per cent had it two to three times a week.[28]

What makes the *ramyŏn* case particularly interesting is the fact that the product is of Japanese origin and entered the Korean diet relatively recently. The prototype of the packaged noodle soup, which could be prepared in a few minutes by just adding hot water, went on sale in Japan in 1958 under the name of Chikin Rāmen. Its inventor, Andō Momofuku (1910–2007), was inspired by the Chinese noodle soup (*shina soba*, nowadays best known as *rāmen*) that had been sold in Japan since the early twentieth century by specialist shops and food peddlers. In Japan the dish experienced a boom twice: first during the 1930s, when the Japanese expansion into Manchuria generated an unprecedented fashion for China, and for a second time during the late 1940s and '50s, when the shortage of rice and American wheat imports compelled the Japanese to rely on noodles as their daily staple.[29]

This second factor played a significant role in the diffusion of instant noodles in South Korea, where, as mentioned above, the government actively stimulated consumption of wheat flour acquired cheaply through the PL 480 aid programme. The Agricultural Trade Development and Assistance Act, commonly known as Public Law No. 480 (PL 480), was passed by the U.S. Congress in 1954 with the purpose of protecting the interests of American farmers by creating markets for their surpluses outside the United States. Park's regime could rely on this source of cheap wheat well into the 1970s, freeing the government from the need to import rice. The volume of U.S. wheat flour imported into South Korea increased from approximately 18,000 tonnes in 1961 to over 100,000 tonnes five years later.[30] The demand continued to rise (from 1,584,000 tonnes in 1975 to 2,648,000 in 1984) even after South Korea had to start importing American wheat at world market prices.[31]

As was the case in Japan, *ramyŏn* played an important role in inculcating wheat consumption among the South Korean population. Already in 1970, instant noodles constituted nearly half (47.2 per cent) of the expenditure of urban families on processed grain products, surpassing other types of noodles, such as *udon*, *naengmyŏn* ('cold noodles') Chinese-style noodles and Italian pasta. By 1985 the share of *ramyŏn* had increased to 74.1 per cent.[32]

A characteristic feature of instant-noodle consumption in South Korea, and a reason for their spectacular sales, is the fact that they are not only consumed at home but can be ordered at canteens and cafeterias. Cooks at these enterprises only need to add hot water before serving them to the customer. Freshly made *ramyŏn* is only served at exclusive Japanese-style *rāmen* restaurants, a far cry from the plebeian

Korean version available at canteens and cafeterias. As Han Kyung-Koo plainly put it, 'Korean-style *ramyeon* started as instant *ramyeon* and has remained so.'[33]

Per capita consumption of wheat in South Korea nearly doubled between 1962 and 2000, rising from 50.7 to 99.0 grams per day. The full magnitude of this transformation comes to light if we consider that the overall consumption of grain in the same period diminished: from 559 grams in 1969 to 310.5 grams per capita per day in 2001.[34] In only seven years, between 1970 and 1977, the GNP per capita increased from U.S.$252 to over $1,000, and more than doubled again a decade later.[35] As the economy kept growing, the dietary adjustments that usually accompany rising standards of living were observed: the ratio of food expenditure to general private consumption expenditure dropped (from 53.8 per cent in 1973 to 42.5 per cent in 1986); the share of the average household budget spent on grain as a percentage of the total food expenditure diminished (from 60 per cent in 1965 to 20.3 per cent in 1990); and per capita consumption of foodstuffs of animal origin such as beef, pork, chicken, eggs, milk and dairy products increased (from 5.5 kg in 1965 to 93.7 kg in 1996), as did consumption of industrially processed foods such as biscuits and commercially prepared meals.

It must be pointed out that these new patterns of consumption developed primarily in urban areas. Farm households, although adjusting to industrialization and the changing pace of life, tended to retain their taste preferences and consumption practices, remaining largely self-sufficient in terms of the production and processing of food. In an account of life in a South Korean fishing and farming village in the late 1960s, Vincent Brandt reports that the bulk of the crop (rice, barley, Chinese cabbage, sweet potatoes, beans, peanuts, wheat, garlic, red chillies, turnip, cucumbers, sesame, flax, corn, kaoliang (sorghum), various spinach-like greens, aubergines and squash) was grown in the village for home consumption, except for small surpluses of peanuts, red chilli, sweet potatoes and garlic, which were sometimes taken to the market town. Brandt notes that even if villagers happened to acquire flour through governmental programmes, they were not particularly fond of it and usually sold it at the market to buy rice.[36]

Another study of South Korean village life, conducted by Clark Sorensen in a farming village of Sangongni, reveals that by the early 1980s some urban consumption patterns had gradually begun to permeate the countryside. 'Although the villagers were still self-sufficient in food staples such as rice, barley and major vegetables,' Sorensen

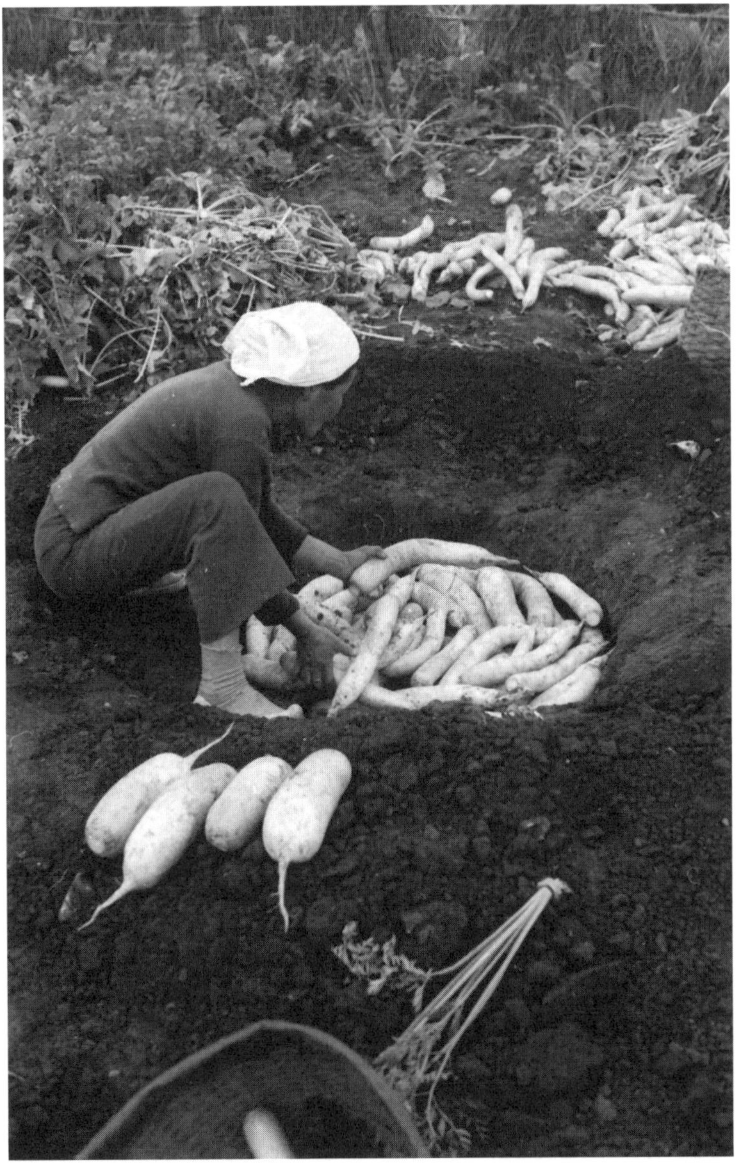

A woman storing radishes in an earthen pit, 1977.

explains, 'other foods such as noodles, liquor, meat, and fruits were regularly purchased at the local periodic markets.'[37] As agricultural productivity dramatically increased after the 1970s (largely owing to governmental programmes of rural revitalization) and self-sufficiency at home could be secured with less land, South Korean farmers were now able to engage in producing cash crops and generating more income. While beer, factory-made noodles and other new items entered their diet, major food-processing practices such as pickling vegetables and making condiments continued in most rural households (see chapter Three). However, with urbanization proceeding at a rapid tempo, by the end of the twentieth century nearly 80 per cent of South Koreans lived in urban areas, more than half of them in the metropolitan cities of Seoul and Pusan.[38] This has meant much more than just a geographic relocation. Of the country's 41 million people, over 27 million lived and worked in social and economic settings that were far removed from those of their parents and grandparents. Their new places of residence made it practically impossible to engage in the home production and processing of staples.[39] The mundane chores of the past have gradually acquired an aura of nostalgia and have become signifiers of a Korean way of life that had been gradually lost under the impact of Japanese colonial rule and the Cold War.

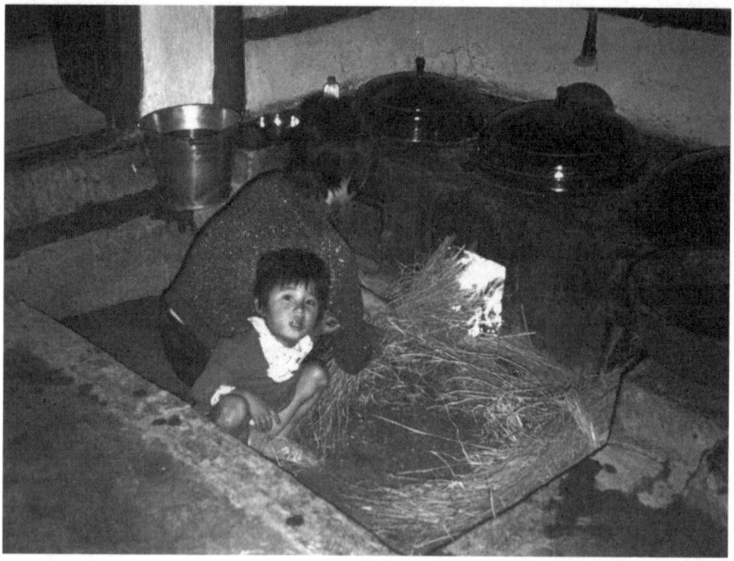

A woman lighting a stove in a rural kitchen, 1971.

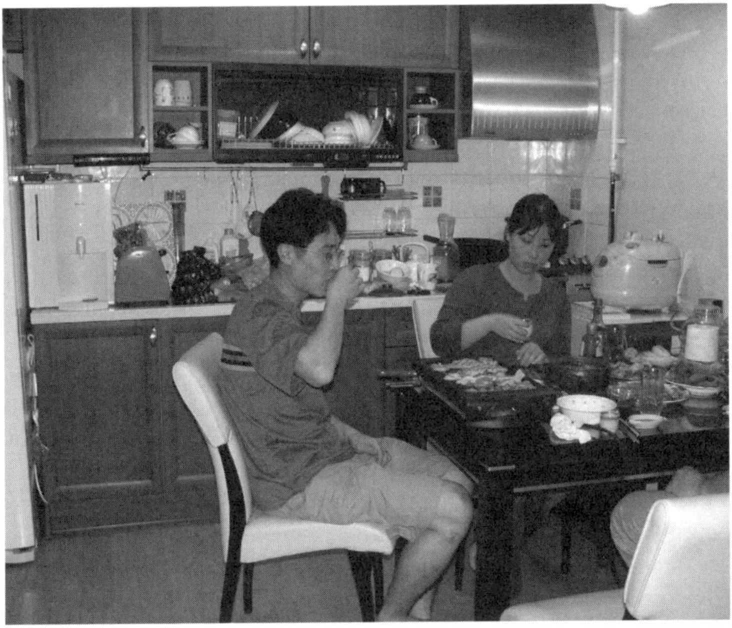

A young couple at mealtime in their urban kitchen, 2003.

The Complex Dilemmas of Affluence

By the 1990s abundance and variety became the key attributes of the South Korean food scene. The majority of its population was able not only to enjoy a diet that in the past had been affordable only to the elite, but to indulge in foreign culinary trends. The multicultural gastronomic scene of half a century earlier was resurrected, and this time the 'colonization' of consumption encompassed the majority of the population.

The economic chaos of the late 1940s, followed by the Korean War, destroyed much of the restaurant culture of colonial Korea (see chapter Two), although top-end establishments continued to operate, patronized by Korean elites and newly arrived Americans. The upmarket restaurant The Grill, which opened at Keijō Railway Station in 1925, now catered to the South Korean political elite, including presidents Syngman Rhee and Park Chung-hee.[40] The majority of Western-style restaurants throughout Seoul were converted into mess halls: Capitol Mess-East, Chosen Mess, Banto Mess, Kirahu Mess, Plaza Hotel Mess, Sheranuhi Hotel Mess, Bizenya Mess, Cho Kwang Mess, Tonga

Mess, Sam Pan Mess, South Korea Mess, Tola Shil Mess, and Nai Ja (Nai Jai) Mess were all originally colonial-era establishments.[41]

While Japanese-style restaurants vanished quickly as their proprietors and patrons repatriated home, Chinese eateries (*Chungguk chip*) steadily increased: from 332 in 1948 to 1,702 ten years later and 2,454 in 1972, the majority operating in the capital.[42] The popularity of Chinese restaurants was greatly sustained by the promotion of flour-based dishes, since noodles and dumplings dominated their menus. These dishes included *udon* noodle soup (in Korean pronounced as *udong*), which had been adopted from the Japanese during the colonial period.

Before the 1980s, when the number of restaurants serving Japanese and Western-style food increased dramatically (see p. 179, Table VIII), the Chinese restaurant remained for ordinary South Koreans the main stage on which to encounter foreign food. The encroachment of American fast food was the most spectacular trend of the 1980s and 1990s. Curiously enough, the very first fast-food store that opened in South Korea, in 1979, was Lotteria – a Japanese replica of McDonald's. The brand had operated in Japan since 1972, a year after the arrival of McDonald's, and was part of the Lotte Group, a large food-processing

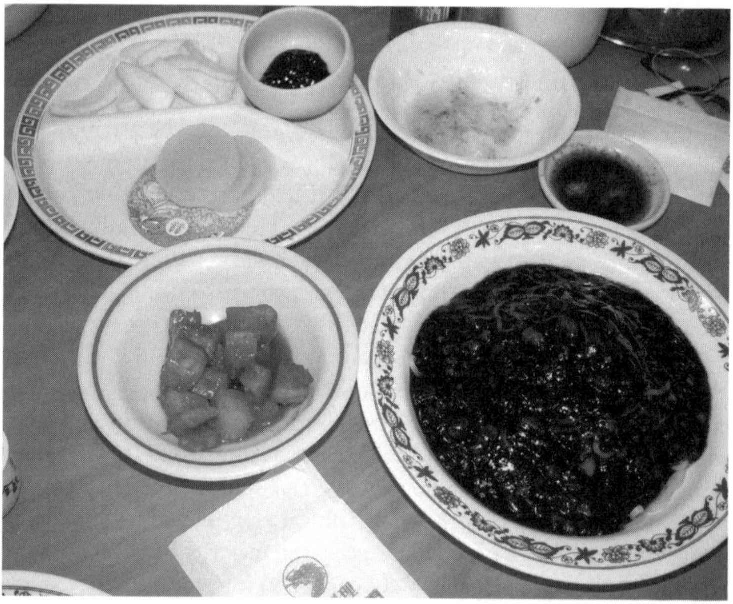

Chajangmyŏn, a signature dish of Chinese restaurants in Korea, served here with radish *kimch'i* and the Japanese-style radish pickle *tanmuji*, 2003.

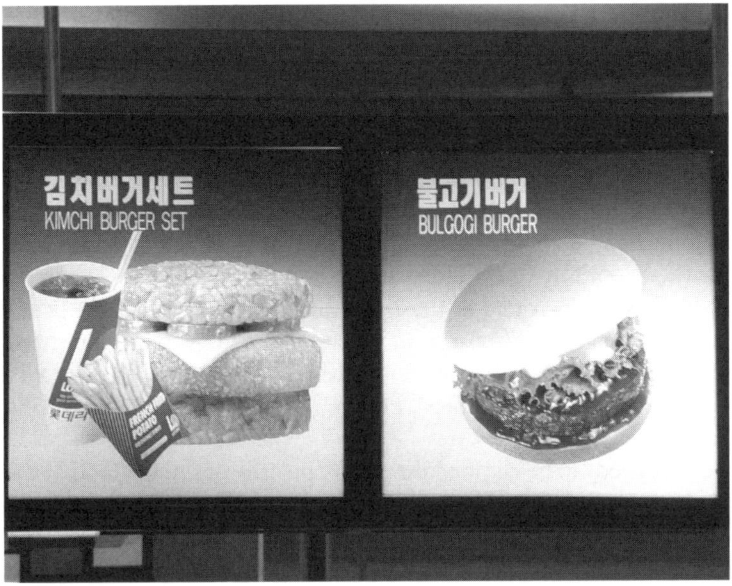

Items designed especially for the Korean market on a menu of the Japanese fast-food chain Lotteria, Seoul, 2003.

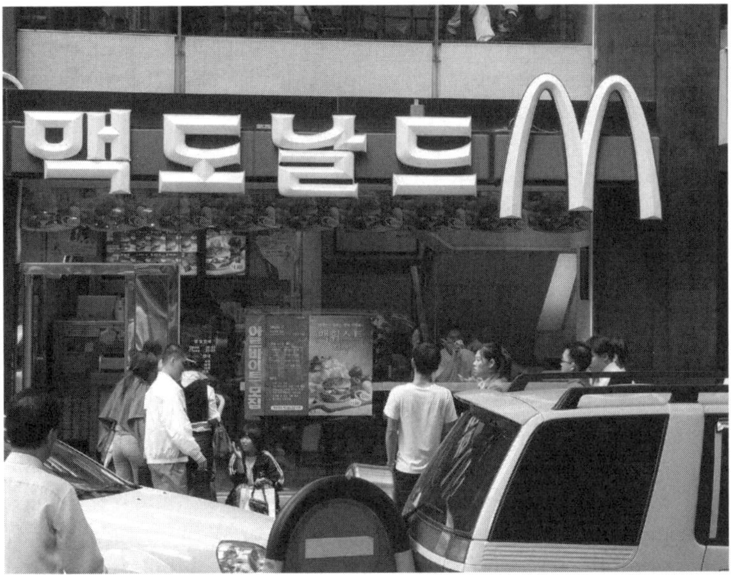

A McDonald's outlet in Seoul, 2003.

conglomerate founded in Japan in 1948 by a first-generation Korean immigrant, Shin Kyŏk-ho (1922–), also known under his Japanese name, Shigemitsu Takeo. The company actively invested in the South Korean food-processing industry soon after the liberalization of South Korean–Japanese relations in 1965, successively increasing its share in the South Korean food market.[43] The major players in the global fast-food industry, such as Burger King, KFC, McDonald's and Pizza Hut, all branched into South Korea during the 1980s, largely in preparation for the Seoul Olympic Games in 1988.[44] As per capita expenditure on dining out increased in the 1980s and early '90s, so did the popularity of foreign food (see p. 179, Tables VIII and IX). By 2001 Lotteria was operating 752 outlets in South Korea, followed by McDonald's (321 outlets), KFC (236 outlets), Popeye's (185 outlets) and Burger King (113 outlets).[45]

It needs to be clarified that the popularity of foreign food at the time remained largely confined within the snack and dining-out categories, and only sporadically featured in home cooking. Even by the end of the twentieth century, with the occasional exception of cooked pasta or Japanese-style instant curry, foreign dishes rarely found their way into Korean kitchens, the 'rice-soup-*kimch'i* pickles-side dishes' pattern (see Introduction) remaining the guiding principle of the majority of Korean meals. Only a handful of foreign dishes managed to establish themselves as components of the established meal pattern. For example, variations of coleslaw often appear as a side dish alongside traditional stews and greens; and various kinds of sausage not infrequently feature on the table, either simply pan-fried, or dipped in flour and egg and then pan-fried (see p. 179, Table X).[46]

Thus the transformation that South Korean consumption practices underwent at the end of the twentieth century manifested itself most profoundly in the culture of dining out.[47] Foreign-style dining stood for affluence and sophistication; it signified the elevation of the South Korean urban culture to the level of multicultural global gastronomy. Yet many Koreans became concerned that the South Korean economy would be adversely affected if they patronized foreign restaurants, and a preference for foreign food was at the time commonly perceived as a sign of conspicuous consumption and vanity, accompanied by fear that, through the consumption of foreign products, 'Korean' culture would fall victim to Japanese or Western infiltration.[48] Along with the recession of the 1990s, this factor might be considered the main reason behind the dramatic slump of Western-style restaurants.

A poster from a *sint'o puri* campaign, 1992.

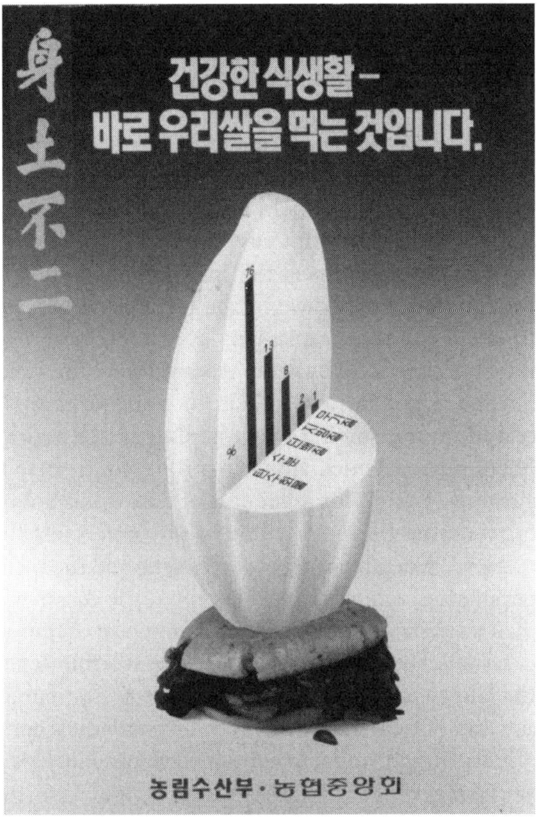
身土不二
건강한 식생활 –
바로 우리쌀을 먹는 것입니다.
농림수산부·농협중앙회

The argument that urban citizens should eat native produce to protect the livelihood of their producer-compatriots in the countryside became increasingly persuasive.

The last point found articulation in 1992 when, facing the introduction of free trade agreements on agricultural products, the National Agricultural Cooperative Federation (Nonghyŏp Chung'anhoe) and the Ministry of Agriculture, Forestry and Fisheries (Nongsin Susanbu) jointly produced a poster promoting the consumption of South Korean agricultural products. The poster's message reads: 'Healthy eating – just eat our rice' and includes the slogan *sint'o puri* (literally 'body and earth are one') in the upper-left corner.[49] The phrase derives from a Buddhist concept of the inseparability of the karma of an individual and that of his/her surroundings. In its popular usage today, *sint'o puri* implies specifically that food from Korean soil is best for Korean bodies.

The publicity that surrounded the various activities of the Agricultural Cooperative Federation undertaken to propagate this idea succeeded in inculcating a common belief among South Korean consumers that food produced in Korea is better tasting and healthier than imported produce. Ironically, as the transformation of consumption patterns continued, South Koreans became increasingly dependent on food imports.

An issue that would in time become a particularly contentious one was the skyrocketing consumption of meat in South Korea and the imports needed to meet the growing demand. Within three decades the consumption of meat in South Korea multiplied by fourteen times, from 6.6 grams per capita per day in 1969 to 91.7 grams in 2001, with the most significant increases recorded since the 1980s: from 13.6 grams in 1980 to 38.8 in 1986, 51.8 in 1992 and 69 grams in 1998.[50] This process of meat assuming a central place in the South Korean diet was a phenomenon which stood in strong contrast to traditional dietary patterns. Except for a handful of elite households, meat-eating had for centuries been a privilege of the uppermost social and economic groups.[51] Korean farmers, who constituted the majority of the Korean population, rarely ate meat except at the summer solstice to keep up their stamina in the oppressive, humid heat of mid-summer, or at ritual occasions, such as household ancestor worship ceremonies (*chesa*).[52] In the late 1970s and early '80s even the richest families in the countryside did not eat meat every day. Moreover, except at banquets, it was rare for an individual to consume even as much as 100 grams of meat at one meal.[53]

Chronic deprivation of meat was the main reason behind the excitement generated by the 'piggie stew' that features in the extract from Ahn Junghyo's novel quoted at the beginning of this chapter. Spam, a branded American canned luncheon meat, became the most emblematic of the food items that entered the Korean diet via military camptowns, primarily because it was perceived as a substitute for meat. For this very same reason, it remained popular long after the role of U.S. military rations as an important source of nutrition disappeared.

Spam has been manufactured from pork shoulder and ham by the Hormel Foods Corporation since 1937. The pink block of fatty, salty processed pork began its life as a symbol of American affluence in the 1940s when it was included in U.S. military canned field rations (C-Rations) and has accompanied the U.S. armed forces at every major combat operation ever since. The quartermasters considered Spam nearly perfect mess-tent food: it was not only nutritious, filling, affordable and shelf-stable, but its rectangular cans were extremely convenient to ship in bulk.[54] Sales increased in the U.S. after the Second World War as many soldiers introduced the product to their families and friends, who had thus far been unfamiliar with it. More importantly, however, Spam became popular in the parts of the world where U.S. troops were stationed. Today the peoples of Guam, South Korea, Okinawa and the Philippines rank as the largest per capita consumers of Spam.[55]

As late as 2003, I experienced the absence of meat from the daily diet at first-hand during a stay at a student boarding house (*hasuk chip*) in the centre of Seoul (see p. 179, Table x). While rice was supplied to students in unlimited quantities at the table of Ms Kim, the proprietor, vegetables constituted the overwhelming majority of side dishes – in the form of *kimch'i*, served raw with a dipping sauce (*ch'ojang*), blanched or pan-fried in batter. Dried baby sardines (*myŏlch'i*) and dried pollack (*pugŏ*) appeared on the table almost daily in various forms. Pan-fried fish and boiled squid were frequently served, too. The absence of meat was the most striking characteristic of the meals served by Ms Kim. Over the course of three months meat was served but rarely, and often in the form of foreign-inspired dishes: minced meat patties (*kogijŏn*), slices of sausage covered in batter and pan-fried (*sosijijŏn*), pieces of wiener sausages fried with onions and strips of fish cake (*odeng*), Japanese-style breaded pork cutlet (*tonkkasŭ*), Japanese-style curry and Western-style hamburgers served with ketchup or soy-based *t'onkkasŭ* sauce. The last three items were clearly intended to appeal to the taste of the student boarders. During my stay at the boarding house I was served grilled meat only once – on the day of my arrival, which I ineptly planned in the middle of Ch'usŏk (Harvest Moon Festival). Since all the other boarders had returned to their parental homes to celebrate the festival, I was allowed to share the festive meal with Ms Kim's family. In short, grilled meat was obviously a treat.

As Ms Kim's Ch'usŏk meal testifies, grilled meat ranks high in the hierarchy of festive dishes, and had by the end of the twentieth century assumed an iconic place in South Korean cuisine, both at home and abroad. *Pulgogi* (thin slices of marinated beef grilled at the table) was selected by the South Korean government as one of the country's representative foods for the 24th Summer Olympic Games in Seoul in 1988, and yet again as one of the key ambassadors in the currently ongoing global promotion of Korean cuisine.

A chief location for the consumption of grilled meat in South Korea is the grilled meat restaurant; these emanate an aura of being the preservers of 'traditional' gastronomic culture in the face of encroaching global trends. While leaning on the longstanding tradition of *nŏbiani kui* – a signature dish of the gentrified classes, made from thick slices of seasoned beef grilled on iron plates over charcoal – the Korean barbecue restaurant is in essence a modern construct.[56] Like Korean restaurant culture itself (see chapter Two), it is a relatively new, twentieth-century phenomenon.

Eateries serving chilled noodle soup (*naengmyŏn*) are considered the first dining establishments to offer on their menus, during the 1930s, a modern version of *nŏbiani kui*. The origins of cookhouses serving inexpensive grilled pork dishes (*twaeji kalbi*, *twaeji pulgogi* and *samgyŏpsal*) are even more recent, dating back to the 1950s.[57] The rich variety of styles of grilling meat – often with specific regional associations – that can currently be sampled at the ubiquitous grilled meat restaurants developed during the last decades of the twentieth century. The best-known examples include *Suwŏn kalbi* (literally, 'ribs from Suwŏn'), which originated from restaurants in the important market town of Suwŏn that attracted both local and itinerant livestock traders, and *I'dong kalbi*, from the region near the city of P'och'ŏn, an area that provided a cross-section of both local and foreign customers due to the presence of military installations.[58] Restaurants in the districts of Tamyang, Haenam, Changhŭng and Kangjin acquired national recognition in lending the names of their respective districts to a style of *kalbi* generically known as *ttŏk kalbi,* taking inspiration from the method of pounding and kneading marinated ribless meat as if it were rice cake dough (*ttŏk*).[59]

In her historical survey of grilled meat restaurants in South Korea, Helen-Louise Brown argues that these establishments were 'conceived in the past and raised in modernity'; in other words, while they offer a genre of food that truly stems from the Korean culinary tradition, it is one that only fully developed in the latter half of the twentieth century. In extension of this argument, I would like to suggest that the Cold War served as the incubating room that nurtured the making of meat into a key symbol of Korean cuisine. In 2003, before the import of U.S. beef was banned in December due to the detection of BSE cases among Washington-state cattle, Korea was the third largest export market for U.S. beef, with annual exports valued at U.S.$1.3 billion.[60]

It was only possible for meat-eating to assume a central place in the Korean diet once imports were liberalized. By 2006 Korea was ranked globally as the sixth largest importer of pork and the seventh

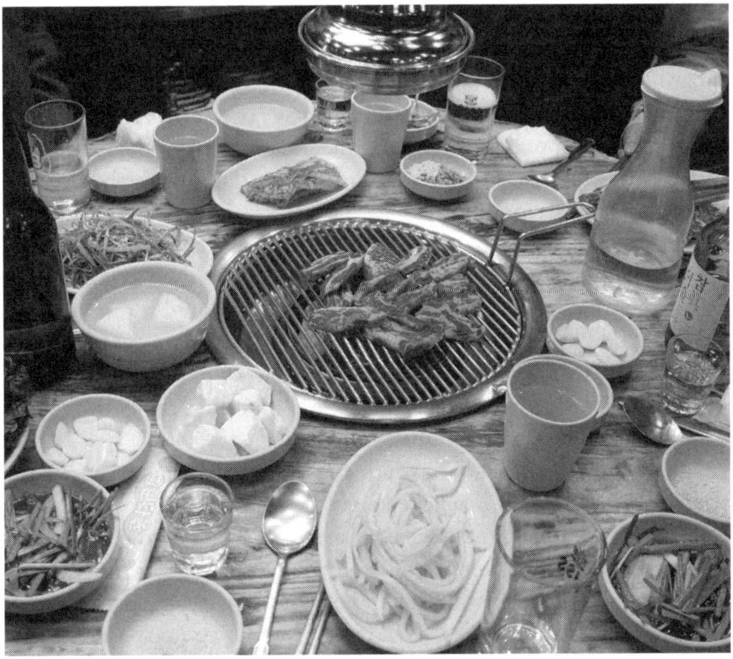

A meal of grilled meat at a traditional restaurant, Seoul, 2003.

largest importer of beef.[61] The irony in the *sint'o puri* movement that promotes the consumption of domestically produced meat, among other measures, lies in the fact that no Korean farm animals are fed with plants produced in Korean soil, but with imported feedstuffs.[62]

Along with the issue of food imports, a major dilemma concerning consumption that developed in South Korea, along with the rising standard of living and rapidly transforming consumption patterns, was the desire to be simultaneously nationalistic and global. The growing ambivalence towards achieving a globalized lifestyle while losing one's Korean identity in the process was largely generated by governmental campaigns directed against *kwasobi* (literally 'excessive consumption') – the term applied to the phenomenon of consuming beyond what was considered appropriate.[63] Campaigns conducted during the late 1980s and early '90s focused on patriotic frugality, warning South Koreans of the dangers inherent in extravagance.

It was by no means a new phenomenon for the South Korean government to advocate frugality and restraint in consumption. The first campaigns date back to the Korean War (see chapter Four) and were successively recycled in the following decades with the blessing of Park Chung-hee himself, who was inspired by similar discourses in Japan.[64] What made the campaign of the 1990s different, however, was the approaching expiration of the image of a prosperous future as the central component of South Korean nationalism. The generation of Koreans who had for decades endured hardship with the promise of future affluence in mind were by the late 1980s ready to measure the return on their sacrifices. Anti-*kwasobi* campaigns expressed a widespread unease about South Korean society. 'The sense of camaraderie built around a shared history of poverty and a shared future of prosperity – albeit never wholly convincing – dissipated as a new generation came of age. This new generation not only had *not* shared the same level of deprivation, it did not share the expectation that the entire nation should sacrifice for a *future* goal.'[65]

Ironically, after 1997, when the Asian financial crisis hit the export-oriented South Korean economy, domestic consumption began to be reconsidered by the policy-makers as the vanguard of the country's economic revitalization. In the post-1997 era, consumer patriotism was no longer defined primarily in term of frugality; consuming itself was elevated to a 'nation-saving act'.[66] Foreign culinary trends were further embraced and diversified, including the booming popularity of Italian, Indian, Thai and other foreign restaurants, as well as the phenomenal success of Starbucks coffee shops and their imitators.[67] However, this consistent encroachment by foreign culinary trends engendered the reassertion of Korean culinary heritage.[68] To eat Korean food became increasingly a matter of conscious decision rather than a habit. In fact, while the number of restaurants serving foreign food in South Korea remained relatively stable between 1993 and 2006 (see p. 179, Table IX), a spectacular growth in restaurants serving Korean food could be observed in the same period – from 151,438 to 261,395 establishments.[69] As Laura Nelson argued in her analysis of South Korean consumer nationalism,

> As South Korean consumers encountered an increasingly complex market, they brought to this context their sense of identification with the nation. At a deeper level, consumers set themselves the larger task of making consumer choices that were in the best interest of the nation – choices that were most 'Korean'.[70]

It is precisely this context that created fertile ground for the dramatic proliferation of Korean-style restaurants and the nostalgic commodification of Korean culinary heritage.

The Food Industry and the Commodification of Tradition

The food industry, together with textiles, played an important role in the South Korean economy before heavy industry emerged during the 1970s. It is extremely difficult to assess the degree of continuity between the colonial food-processing enterprises (see chapter One) and their post-liberation descendants. Clear connections in terms of investment and the entrepreneurship of the Korean business elite have been traced and documented by Dennis McNamara, who found 'postcolonial continuities most striking in patterns of concentration, continued prominence of the family in large-scale enterprise and persistence of close-business-state ties'.[71] Pak Hŭng-sik (the founder of Hwasin Department Store) and Kim Yŏn-su (joint investor in Shōwa Kirin Beer Company) were during the 1960s closely involved in developing South Korean flour and sugar manufacture, as well as in the export of ginseng, vegetable gelatine and marine products to Hong Kong and Macao. Kim's Samyang concern (*chaebŏl*), which maintained close ties with Japan, stood behind the manufacture of *ramyŏn*.[72]

The devastation of the Korean War destroyed most production facilities and machinery, but we may surmise that, as in the case of soy sauce manufacture (see chapter Three), the know-how and experience that Korean employees acquired on the job was to a certain extent utilized during the 1950s and '60s. According to the statistics of the Home Ministry, 1,068 food-processing enterprises and 898 beverage manufacturers were registered by the autumn of 1955 in Seoul and its surroundings.[73] Another governmental source lists three sugar refineries, 156 *kanjang* and *toenjang* manufacturers, and 1,300 factories producing confectionery (*kwaja kongjang*) operating in South Korea as of 1955.[74] The *Year Book of Public Health and Social Statistics 1961* records 687 cake manufacturers, 396 bakeries and 49 cider and lemonade factories, which might suggest a slight consolidation of the industry.[75] An economic white paper for 1962 provides us with more detailed statistics on canneries, whose production was primarily exported and contracted by the government as rations for the armed forces.[76]

Like the entire South Korean economy, the 1960s marked a turning point for the food-processing industry, as it was becoming increasingly stimulated by the state-geared economic plans and the Vietnam War. Between 1960 and 1984 the growth ratio in terms of added value increased by 10.5 per cent, 2.5 per cent higher than the GNP growth rate.[77] Between 1976 and 1986 the production value increased seven times, with sectors such as meat processing and dairy experiencing spectacular growth (see p. 180, Table XI).

Unlike during the Korean War (see chapter Four), when ROK soldiers were provided with special combat rations produced in Japan, at the time of the Vietnam War it was the turn of the South Korean food industry to cash in. South Korean soldiers deployed to Vietnam could from 1966 onwards rely on the shipment of rations from home, which for the very first time included canned *kimch'i* pickles especially developed for this purpose.[78] Soldiers were the first consumers of canned *kimch'i*, followed during the 1970s by Korean construction workers in the Middle East. The *kimch'i* processing industry began to truly thrive after the 1980s, when the Korean pickle was exported to foreign markets for consumption by non-Koreans.[79] The product did particularly well in Japan: between 1990 and 2000 the import of Korean *kimch'i* increased nearly tenfold, from 3,432 to 30,000 tonnes.[80]

The popularity of *kimch'i* in Japan greatly stimulated the South Korean *kimch'i* processing industry. Ironically, it was Japanese attempts to capitalize on manufacturing *kimch'i* that inflamed Korean claims to its 'ownership'. This dispute, commonly known as the 'Kimch'i War' (*kimch'i chŏnjaeng*), began in 1996 when Japan proposed designating *kimuchi* (the Japanese pronunciation of *kimch'i*) an official Atlanta Olympic food. By then Japanese–Korean trade relations were already under stress due to the fact that Japan had already been involved in exporting the Japanese 'instant' version of *kimch'i*, which lacked the distinctive flavour deriving from the fermentation process. In response, South Korea had filed a case with the Codex Alimentarius Commission (CAC), part of the United Nations Food and Agriculture Organization, arguing that there was a need to establish an international *kimch'i* standard.[81] In September 2000 the 20th Session of the Codex Committee on Processed Fruits and Vegetables advanced the Draft Standard for Kimchi for final adoption, which took place on 5 July 2001. The decision was interpreted by the Korean press as a failure on the part of Japan to challenge Korea with its poor *kimch'i* imitation.[82]

Kimch'i does not seem to be an isolated case. Success in the Japanese market seems to be setting the stage for national recognition, followed by efforts towards commodification and global promotion, for a number of Korean products. One of the most recent examples is *makgŏlli*, a milky alcoholic beverage made by fermenting rice, wheat and water. Originally a poor man's drink – it is also known under the name of *nongju* ('farmer's liquor') – *makgŏlli* has since 2009 enjoyed a true renaissance, and is served at high-end *makgŏlli*-themed bars and posh restaurants.[83] What makes the *makgŏlli* revival particularly interesting is the fact that it was the Japanese, not Koreans, who 'rediscovered' the drink. The enormous popularity of *makgŏlli* in Japan received wide coverage in the South Korean media, sparking the interest of Korean consumers. Total exports of *makgŏlli* in 2011 more than doubled in comparison to 2010, with some 92 per cent destined for Japan.[84] As was the case with *kimch'i*, a healthy image played a critical role in stimulating Japanese interest in *makgŏlli*. Its alleged ability to increase longevity, lower cholesterol, reduce blood pressure and boost the immune system began to be emphasized in Korea as well, aided by nostalgia for the Korean lifestyle of the past which had been lost on the way to economic affluence. These themes were also central to the advertising strategies of *makgŏlli* manufacturers on home ground.

As the case of *makgŏlli* indicates, the nostalgia market for romanticized versions of the past, represented by goods, performances and experiences associated with a vanished way of life – including food and drink – has been rapidly growing in South Korea since the late 1990s.[85] As elsewhere, it is stimulated by a longing for an imagined cultural authenticity in the face of being disappointed by the promises of consumer society to fulfil our commodified desires.[86] In parallel with similar developments elsewhere,[87] this rediscovery of Korea's own culinary heritage follows a period of rapid economic growth and increasing familiarity – even infatuation – with foreign food. The Seoul Olympics of 1988 and the political liberalization of the following years marked the beginning of the rapidly growing exposure of the South Korean population to foreign culinary trends. However, largely influenced by the government campaigns directed towards curbing conspicuous consumption, South Koreans experienced a dilemma between the urges to be nationalistic and global. 'In a manner everywhere conducive to nostalgia, South Koreans express anxiety over the corrupting influence of new wealth', writes Laurel Kendall, a leading anthropologist of Korea, in a recently published volume that tackles the consumption of various forms of Korean commodified tradition.[88]

The Asian financial crisis of 1997 and the tight fiscal reforms required in return for a rescue package offered by the International Monetary Fund brought about inflation, wage cuts and reduced consumer spending. These developments functioned as a powerful stimulant for the nostalgic expropriation of traditional values, including the growing appreciation for Korean food. This trend was further reinforced by the revival of the lavish and formal style of dining served at the court of the Chosŏn Dynasty (1392–1910) – commonly known today under the name *kungjung ŭmsik*, translated into English as 'Korean Royal Cuisine'.

The Royal Cuisine of the Chosŏn Royal Court (Chosŏn Wangjo Kungjung Ŭmsik), as this Important Intangible Cultural Asset No. 38 is officially labelled, was transmitted in its present form through Han Hui-sun (1889–1972), the last surviving court lady responsible for the preparation of the king's meals.[89] The 'Important Intangible Cultural Asset' (Chungyo Muhyŏng Munhwajae, IICA) system was founded by the South Korean government in 1962 with the aim of fostering national pride through the promotion and careful portrayal of specific aspects of Korea's history and culture. The system supports theatrical forms, music, handicrafts, martial arts and anything else deemed 'historically valuable'.[90] By 1985 there were 83 genres recognized as IICAs and 200 individuals had been appointed to safeguard the transmission of the IICAs, the so-called 'holders' (*poyuja*), more commonly referred to as Human Cultural Assets (In'gan Munhwajae). These 'holders' are required to perform and teach their art, and since 1968 they have been provided with a monthly stipend to aid their activities. To encourage and support the study of IICAs, the government also gives financial support to promising students who will at some point take over.[91]

Han was appointed the Human Cultural Asset No. 77 in 1971, at the age of 83. Following her death a year later, her disciple Hwang Hye-sŏng (1920–2006) took over the task. Unlike Han, Hwang had not been a royal cook herself, but began studying the secrets of the royal kitchen from Han in 1943, soon after completing her education in the home economics department of Kyōto Joshi Senmon Gakkō (currently Kyoto Women's University) in Japan. This background proved useful in researching and recording the culinary practices of the Korean court, from its recipes and table setting to protocol and terminology. Hwang Hye-sŏng was in fact the one who actively lobbied to have *kungjung ŭmsik* designated as an IICA by the government. After her death, she was replaced in the role of Human Cultural Asset No. 77 by her daughter Han Pong-nyŏ, who currently holds the title.[92]

The commercialization of royal court cuisine began in the early 1990s, when the Hwang family began to expand its activities beyond lectures and publications. In 1991 the Hwangs opened the restaurant Chihwaja, inside the National Theatre, and began selling exclusive Chihwaja-brand confectionery and snacks.[93] In 2002 Han Pong-nyŏ worked closely with Asiana Airlines to develop a royal cuisine menu for its first-class passengers and during the following year supervised cooking on the set of the celebrated TV series *Taejanggŭm* ('Jewel in the Palace'); this was to be broadcast on the South Korean MBC channel from September onwards. The drama depicted the life story of a sixteenth-century historical character, a female who combined the career of royal chef with that of the king's private physician. Since intrigues and struggles for power in the highly stratified (all-female) royal kitchen constituted the core of the plot, cooking scenes featured prominently throughout the story.

The series was broadcast twice a week, each Monday and Tuesday, at the prime-time slot of 9:55 to 10:55 p.m. The viewing rate rose at a spectacular rate, from 19 per cent at the time of the second episode to 28 per cent two weeks later, and surpassed an astonishing 50 per cent by mid-November. Every week millions of South Korean viewers were becoming acquainted with the half-imagined tradition of cooking and eating at the Royal Court. By the time the show ended in March 2004, *Taejanggŭm* was declared the most popular historical drama ever aired on Korean television, and *kungjung ŭmsik* was transformed into an article of mass consumption.

Because of the popularity of the series, the exclusive royal cuisine was turned into a nationwide obsession. Department stores and restaurants immediately responded to the new fashion. During the second weekend of November, for example, when the viewing rate of the drama began to approach 50 per cent, the Lotte Department Store in Seoul organized in its underground food hall a mini-exhibition of royal cuisine featuring menus served at the restaurant Chihwaja, managed by the Hwang family. From late November to mid-December the upmarket Seoul restaurant Fountain Plaza treated its customers, next to the regular buffet menu, to a wide selection of royal dishes. During the following months the *Taejanggŭm* soundtrack could often be heard as piped music at upmarket food halls and supermarkets.[94]

Numerous housewives in Seoul signed up for cooking classes at Hwang's Institute of Royal Cuisine (Kungjung Ŭmsik Yŏng'uwŏn). The institute had been giving lessons in royal cuisine for decades, but in the autumn of 2003 it had to hire additional instructors and renovate its premises in order to accommodate the crowds of students. The first set of cookery books and cooking videos featuring the main actress from the *Taejanggŭm* series accompanied by the country's leading culinary expert went on sale in January 2004.[95]

As the highest authority on royal cuisine and its ambassador at home and abroad, Hwang and her family had considerable power over the process of 'defining, formalizing and standardizing royal court cuisine', effectively monopolizing its branding and commodification. As Okpyo Moon argues in her excellent analysis of the royal cuisine revival in South Korea, defining and understanding the royal cuisine solely on the basis of Han Hui-sun's memories and their reproduction by Hwang and her descendants is problematic. 'The concept requires a more systematic redefinition on the basis of thorough research that traces its evolution.'[96]

Moon's scepticism concerning the authenticity of Korean royal cuisine notwithstanding, this newly invented part of Korean culinary heritage is now ready to be exported abroad. Exclusive restaurants serving *kungjung ŭmsik* also provide contemporary South Koreans with an opportunity to engage in conspicuous consumption while remaining comfortable with their nationalist consciences.

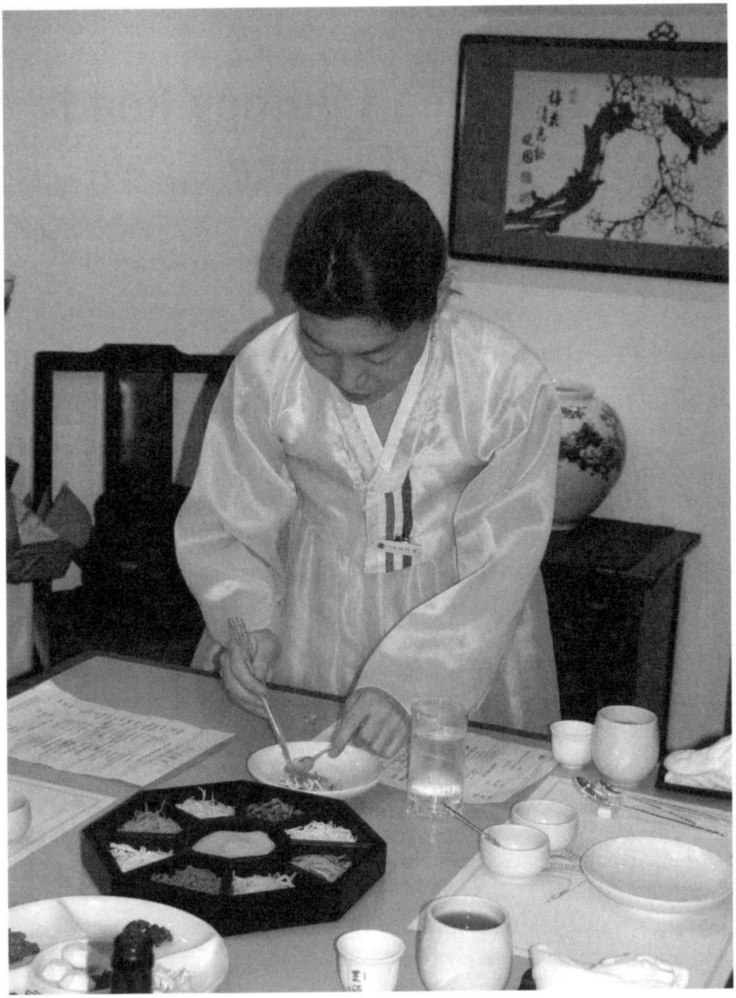

A waitress dressed in a traditional Korean dress (*hanbok*) serving one of the courses at Chihwaja restaurant, 2003.

6
North Korea's Bumpy Road to Affluence

The Restaurant Boom in Pyongyang

At about the same time that South Koreans launched the global campaign for the promotion of Korean cuisine, their northern neighbours were becoming familiar with American fast food. In October 2009 the international media reported on the very first fast-food outlet in downtown Pyongyang, which had opened a few months earlier under the name Samtaesong (literally 'three big stars').[1] The second outlet followed in October 2010 in Kaseon Youth Park, a relic of the 1980s cultural exchange with Russia in downtown Pyongyang.

In contrast to South Korea, Japan, Hong Kong, Taiwan and China, where the leading brands of the global fast-food industry, such as KFC and McDonald's, were the ones that introduced citizens to the American way of dining,[2] the first fast-food outlet in North Korea was modelled on a relatively unknown local company from Virginia: Waffletown USA. In addition to the standard fast-food menu of hamburgers, french fries, fried chicken and hot dogs, Samtaesong in Pyongyang sells Belgian waffles, the signature item of the Waffletown brand. Despite the similarities, the management stresses that the concept and menu have merely been 'borrowed', and that Samtaesong is not a Waffletown franchise.[3]

The man in charge of this pioneering fast-food chain in North Korea is Singapore entrepreneur Patrick Soh, who holds the franchise rights for Waffletown in Asia and has successfully operated two outlets in Singapore since 2006.[4] The two main investors in the business are Quek Chek Lan, managing director of the Aetna Group, which has been trading with the North Koreans in metal and minerals for more than 25 years, and his business associate Timothy Tan. The three set up Sinpyong International to invest in North Korea, and next to Samtaesong have plans for a Western-style beer garden and a supermarket.

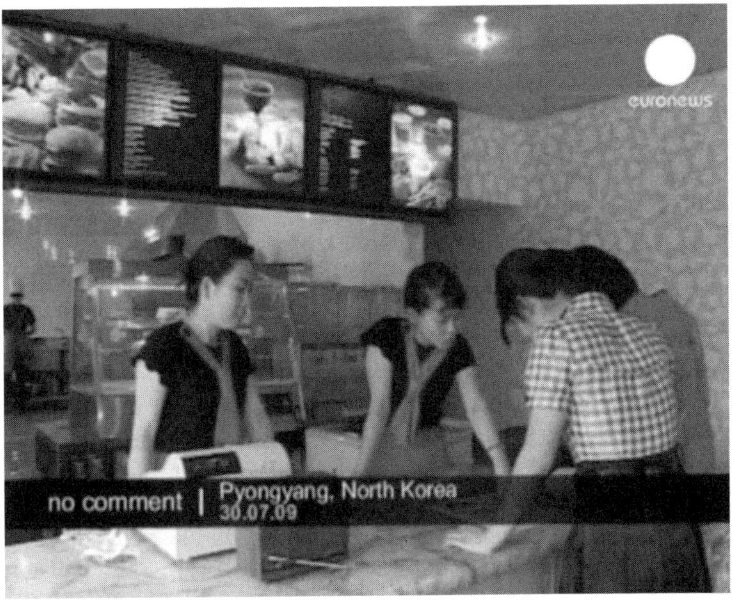

Screenshot from a documentary introducing the first North Korean fast-food restaurant, Samtaesong.

It seems at first sight surprising to find the epitome of the American culture of consumption at the heartland of a Stalinist regime. The connection appears less striking when placed in the perspective of the Soviet infatuation with hamburgers in the early 1940s, following the much-publicized excursion to the United States of the Soviet minister for the food industry, Anastas Mikoyan. While touring the U.S. in the summer of 1936, he was so impressed by the efficiency of hamburgers that he decided to bring them home. Within a couple of years hamburgers were being manufactured in the Soviet Union using imported American machinery, and hot dog and hamburger stands operated on the streets of Moscow. Plans were made to increase production by 27 times by 1942 in accordance with the third Five Year Plan.[5] Standardized and cheap American fast food, along with other products of the American food industry such as cornflakes, ice-cream and ketchup, fitted very well with the dominant mode of thinking regarding goods in Stalin's Russia.

Although the parallels with the Russian hamburger experiment are striking, the opening of a fast-food restaurant in Pyongyang has been motivated by different goals. The overwhelming majority of the

North Korean population cannot afford to dine at Samtaesong, even on special occasions. As Korea specialist Andrei Lankov reports in his collection of essays on daily life in North Korea, the over 500 restaurants that Pyongyang counted in 2005 catered mainly to three kinds of customers: foreigners, North Korean nouveau-riche entrepreneurs and members of the North Korean political establishment.[6] The second and third categories were becoming increasingly intertwined, as by that time a market economy was acquiring a firm foothold in North Korea.

Following the collapse of the planned economy during the 1990s, a true outburst of entrepreneurial spirit took place, in particular after the 'Market Stimulation Measures' announced by North Korean authorities in March 2003. The number of people involved in making handmade goods, trading in markets and other small-scale businesses drastically increased. The North Korean authorities not only gave small-scale commercial and industrial businesses tacit permission to operate, but began to profit from these new activities. The most well-known example was the introduction of 'market use fees' – de facto tax-like payments – for vendors in the ever-expanding markets.[7] In her award-winning book *Nothing to Envy: Real Lives in North Korea*, Barbara Demick retells the stories of North Korean defectors who were compelled to trade at these markets in order to survive. One of her interviewees recalls her mother, Mrs Song, selling homemade tofu and imitation ice-cream made by flavouring the milky water that was left over from tofu making with red beans and sugar, and freezing it. Later she took up selling homemade cookies, but as the testimony below demonstrates, the life of North Korean petit-entrepreneurs like Mrs Song was far from easy.[8]

> Mrs Song got up at 5:00 a.m. to do the baking. The competition was stiff and her cookies needed to be fresh. She didn't have a cart or even a crate from which to sell her product, so she put the cookies in a plastic basin that she would carry wrapped on her back like a baby until she got to a main street with a lot of pedestrians and not too many competitors. She hung around markets and the big square in front of the train station. . . . [At] the end of a fourteen-hour workday, she had about 100 won – 50 cents – in her pocket, and a few bags of other goods, sometimes red peppers or a few lumps of coal, that she took in exchange for cookies. It was just enough for her to buy food for dinner and the ingredients for the next batch of cookies . . .

> Thousands of middle-aged women were doing much the same thing as Mrs Song.[9]

While food stalls and markets catered to the North Korean masses, the restaurant business targeted at the elites and foreign visitors experienced a genuine boost, especially in the capital and around tourist destinations. In March 2009 the magazine *Uriminjokkiri* ('Our Nation by Itself') – the primary mouthpiece of North Korean propaganda on the Internet – proudly announced that eighteen restaurants in Pyongyang's prime restaurant district situated near the Koryo Hotel had been renovated.[10] Even before this facelift took place, English-language travel guides to North Korea remarked on the improvements in Pyongyang's dining scene in the late 2000s. An edition of Bradt's travel guide from 2008 begins its 'Where to Eat?' section as follows: 'Pyongyang is far removed from being London or Bangkok, but bars and restaurants are opening all the time and it is a long, long way from the Pyongyang of not-very-old-at-all.'[11] Along with establishments offering traditional Korean meals, the North Korean capital nowadays boasts places where one can get Western, Japanese and Chinese food. The North Korea section of the Lonely Planet guide to Korea of 2007 highly recommends Pyolmuri (aka Galaxy or Constellation) for serving 'good coffee' and 'delightful' cakes and pies. Pyolmuri was the first to sell pizza, pasta, hamburgers and cocktails in the North Korean capital,[12] but the competition tightened with the opening of Samtaesong in 2009 and an Italian restaurant (Ittaria Ryori Chŏnmun Siktang, literally 'a restaurant specializing in Italian cuisine') a year earlier. The latter received lengthy attention on North Korean state television, and the feature is now available for the whole world to watch on YouTube.[13]

The new dining trends are additions to the existent, although modest, North Korean restaurant tradition. Two establishments that have for decades defined the gastronomic landscape of socialist Pyongyang are the restaurants Okryugwan (*ongnyugwan* literally translates as 'Jade Stream Pavilion') and Ch'ŏngnyugwan ('Pure Stream Pavilion'). Both are prime examples of typical 'mass restaurants', with several dining halls and banqueting rooms that can seat up to 2,000 people. Unlike dining establishments that cater exclusively to the needs of foreigners, both Okryugwan and Ch'ŏngnyugwan are open to North Koreans as well. As Lankov explains, in the past, tickets for entry to such restaurants used to be distributed through work units or other connections, but these days they are on sale to anyone who is able to pay for them.[14]

Okryugwan, which has been in operation since 1960, is recognized as the major guardian of the North Korean culinary tradition. It is particularly well known for its cold noodles (*naengmyŏn*), the most celebrated dish of the North. However, when in the summer of 2009 the restaurant was featured in the very first restaurant commercial ever aired on North Korean television, it did not advertise noodles but quail dishes (*mech'uri ryori*). The advert encouraged potential customers to try Okryugwan's quail menu – praised as 'delicious and nourishing' and a rich source of vitamins B1, B2, B6, B12, PP and E – which would be on offer from 1 September.[15] It was aired alongside a rather lengthy advert for Taedonggang beer. Production of this North Korean beer brand began in April 2002 in the plant that had formerly belonged to Britain's Usher's brewery in Wiltshire, which had ceased operations two years earlier. The brewery was taken apart, shipped piece by piece to Pyongyang and reassembled under the banner of the Taedonggang Beer Factory, named after a river that runs through the capital.[16]

Adverts for both beer and quail dishes appeared on North Korean television in the summer of 2009, but were soon abruptly discontinued, allegedly due to the interference of Kim Jong-il himself.[17] Annalists speculate that the TV advert issue reveals tensions between the Great Leader and his top media advisor Cha Sung-su.[18] Nonetheless, regardless of the relatively short shelf-life of the ads, the fact that they were produced and aired in the first place confirms the general direction of North Korean consumer culture at the dawn of the twenty-first century

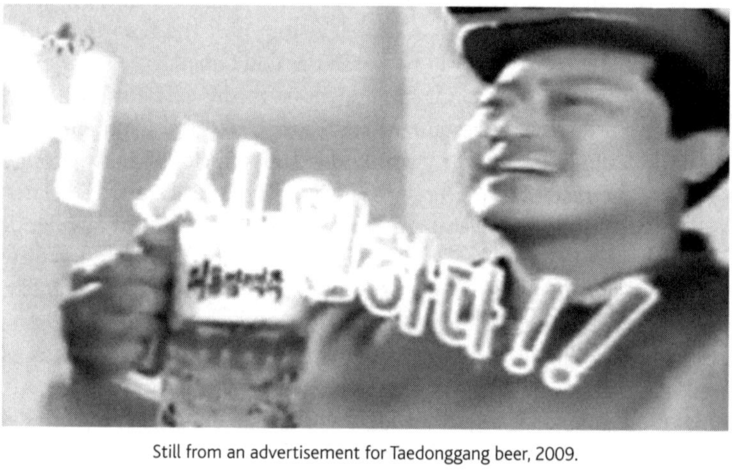

Still from an advertisement for Taedonggang beer, 2009.

The bottle label of the North Korean beer brand Pyongyang.

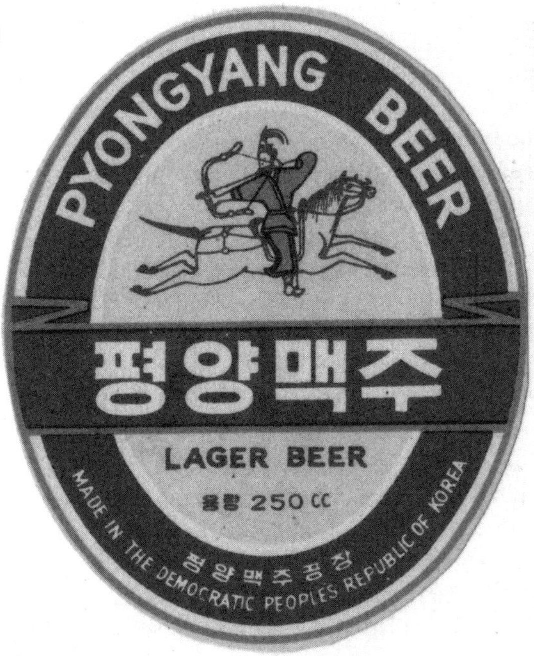

– towards an apprehensive yet consecutive embrace of the principles and practices of the market economy.

The Famine of the 1990s

While events such as the opening of the Samtaesong outlet or the Taedonggang beer advertisement occasionally produce international headlines, they are incapable of overshadowing a very different theme that, along with the nuclear programme, has dominated news reporting about North Korea since the mid-1990s: the famine. The dire food shortages have not only become a potent symbol of North Korea's economic collapse, but a forceful emblem of the regime's violation of human rights.

The food shortage in North Korea gained worldwide attention in 1995 when the North Korean government appealed for humanitarian food aid to the United Nations. The UN agricultural assessment published in December that year reported a food deficit in North Korea amounting to nearly 50 per cent of the food requirement for the entire population – a figure greater than the one that had caused the Ethiopian famine ten years earlier.[19] However, because of a lack of transparency and other problems in the working relationship with the DPRK government, the aid agencies exercised caution in classifying the North Korean food crisis as a 'famine'. Expressions such as 'grave food supply problems', 'on the knife edge of famine' and 'famine in slow motion' were customarily used. This last term proves particularly helpful for understanding the nature of the North Korean famine. According to the economic historian Suk Lee, who conducted an extensive assessment of the famine, the most characteristic feature of this humanitarian disaster was the fact that instead of eruptive demographic losses occurring over relatively short periods of time, the entire population got gradually but persistently weaker.[20] The famine is presumed to have reduced the average life expectancy in North Korea from 66.8 years in 1993 to 60.4 years in 2001.[21]

While estimates of the death toll of the North Korean famine range from a few hundred thousand up to 2 million, the most trustworthy assessment indicates that there were 688,000 excess deaths between 1 January 1994 and 31 August 1999, which translates to 0.53 per cent of the total population.[22] The figure appears relatively modest in comparison to the major twentieth-century famines such as the Chinese 'Great Leap Forward' famine of 1958–62 that killed 30–33 million people, or the Cambodian famine of 1979 that wiped out 1.5 to 2 million people in just one year.[23] The death toll of the North Korean famine seems particularly low if one considers its rather prolonged duration. The climax of the crisis took place in the five-year period between 1994 and 1999, which followed a six-year period of considerably curtailed food supply. The relatively small population loss and the prolonged period of famine are considered the two basic features of the DPRK famine.

For international aid agencies, an additional peculiarity of the North Korean setting was the fact that they were not allowed to develop independent channels for delivering food to the people, but had to rely on the state Public Distribution System (PDS).[24] North Korean authorities were in total control of where to distribute the available food and when, shifting the food aid to different areas, so that as few people as possible would starve. While this strategy resulted in a relatively low level of demographic loss, it was achieved at the cost of a severe health risk that is likely to haunt the North Korean population for decades to come. Because the severe food shortages continued for so long, it is predicted that extensive damage has been inflicted on the development of an entire generation of North Korean children. Medical specialists agree that the consequences of malnutrition experienced in the growth period include not just immediate adverse effects such as decreased immune function and the subsequent rise of mortality rates, but also long-term effects such as reduced work capacity and impaired cognitive, emotional and social functions.[25] According to the assessment of the U.S. National Intelligence Council, by 2009–2013 up to one-third of potential North Korean military conscripts might have cognitive deficiencies that disqualify them for service.[26]

Such projections seem largely overstated, but anthropometric data acquired through surveys conducted by the United Nations in 1997 confirms the gravity of the situation. The three anthropometric parameters for the evaluation of nutritional status are the weight-for-age (WAZ), weight-for-height (WHZ) and height-for-age (HAZ) scores calculated for each child. While a low WHZ score signifies acute malnutrition, a low HAZ score is a major indicator of chronic malnutrition.[27] In other words, a child's height exposes important information about his or her biological welfare during a prolonged period of time, while weight merely indicates short-term conditions.[28] The nutritional survey of North Korean children taken in 1997 confirmed that while only 16 per cent of the children aged between six months and seven years were acutely malnourished (wasted), 62 per cent were suffering from chronic undernutrition (stunting).[29] Based on this data, it was estimated that by the age of seven North Korean children were at least 12 cm shorter than South Korean children.[30] Since North and South Koreans were only relatively recently separated politically into two populations, it is very unlikely that genetic influences caused this difference.

It goes without saying that the U.S.$2.3 billion of international humanitarian aid that poured into the country between 1995 and 2005 saved the North Korean population from mass-scale starvation.[31] The World Food Programme (WFP) – an umbrella organization falling under the United Nations that distributes aid provided by the governments of UN members – functioned as the key channel for humanitarian assistance and the chief negotiator with the North Korean government on behalf of the humanitarian community.[32] Bilateral aid, mainly from South Korea, Japan and China, came second in importance, and was followed by the NGO sector, consisting of various non-profit organizations such as the International Federation of the Red Cross, Caritas and a variety of local organizations, primarily from South Korea and Japan.[33]

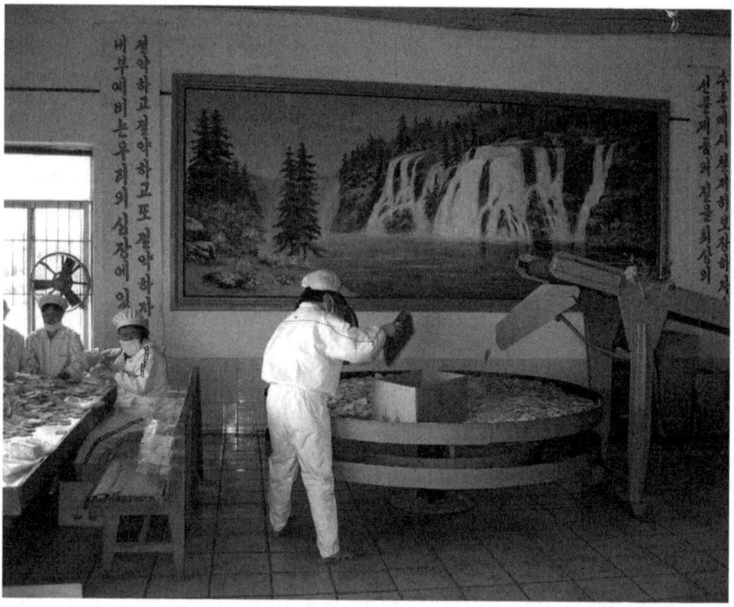
절약하고 절약하고 또 절약하자
내부예비는 우리의 심장에 있

One of the factories making fortified biscuits run by the World Food Programme in North Korea, 2008.

At the outset of the humanitarian operation in North Korea, the incoming food was comprised mainly of cereals, pulses and beans. When nutritional surveys revealed extremely high levels of malnutrition among children, providing more easily digestible food for children under the age of six and pregnant and nursing mothers became the core activity of WFP in North Korea. Local production of foods fortified with minerals and vitamins began in May 1999, expanding to nineteen factories by the end of the WFP emergency operation in 2005.[34] A variety of so-called 'fortified blended foods' (FBF) – mixtures of grains, soybeans, pulses, oilseeds and dried skimmed milk fortified with vitamins and minerals – form the basis of the food aid operations by the WFP throughout the world. In North Korea, Rice Milk Blend (RMB) was provided to the youngest children in orphanages and paediatric hospitals and wards. Corn Soy Milk Blend (CSM) and Cereal Milk Blend (CMB) were offered at orphanages, nurseries and kindergartens, as well as to pregnant and nursing mothers. In accordance with the WFP principle of adapting food aid to local diets, the blends were cooked into a Korean-style porridge (*chuk*), either plain or mixed with boiled sweet potato (*koguma yŏngyangjuk*) or fried vegetables (*kamja yŏngyangjuk*, *hobak yŏngyangjuk*). Fortified corn flour was utilized in sweet potato pancakes (*koguma chijimi*).[35] Vitamin-fortified biscuits were delivered to primary schools and fortified noodles to malnourished mothers. The WFP logo was stamped on the biscuits in an attempt to prevent the food from being used for unintended purposes and/or undeserving recipients.

Despite all these efforts, the problem of child malnutrition remained high in North Korea. The assessment conducted in October 2004 confirmed that 37 per cent of children under the age of six examined in this assessment were stunted, 23 per cent were underweight and 7 per cent were wasted.[36] Moreover, the DPRK Government began in early 2008 to publicly acknowledge that the country was again facing food shortages due to the destruction caused by the August 2007 floods and the low harvest output of the 2007–8 season. A WFP Emergency Operation for North Korea was launched in September 2008, initially for fifteen months, but was then extended to the end of June 2010.[37]

Since the famine itself is not the focus of this chapter, I will not elaborate on it further. Extensive literature on it is available in English that offers an exhaustive source of information on the causes and effects of the famine, the international aid efforts and their diplomatic consequences.[38] The famine is important in the narrative of this volume because it is in such striking juxtaposition to the dietary affluence of the South and because it marks the turning point in the economic, social and political development of North Korea. No other event since the establishment of the DPRK in 1948 has had such a striking impact. Human tragedy aside, the request for humanitarian aid in the mid-1990s has opened the country to the penetration, however restricted, of capitalist influence. The crumbling of the Public Distribution System led to the loosening of state control over the population, as well as depriving the state of the monopoly of food production and trade. Along with a humanitarian disaster, the famine of the 1990s brought about a monumental social and economic change in North Korea, turning the country into a mixture of the worst elements of the two economic systems: the socialist inefficiencies of production and the crudeness of market principles. Today this schizophrenic reality divides Korean society into those with access to consumer goods and those leading a hand-to-mouth existence on the verge of starvation. The famine serves as a watershed in North Korean history, a symbolic divide between life in a socialist paradise and the harsh reality of a system in transition.

Who Is to Blame?

In the official explanation offered by the North Korean regime, the famine was attributed to two major causes: natural disasters and the decline in preferential trade relations with Russia and China. The 'fraternal' aid that the country received from the USSR and China for decades placed North Korea in a very vulnerable position once both states transformed from a command to a market economy in the early 1990s and began to demand market prices for their exports. For example, the chemical fertilizer on which North Korean agriculture was heavily dependent could not be manufactured without the import of petrochemical feedstock from Russia.[39]

Stephan Haggard and Marcus Noland, two prominent U.S. analysts of the North Korean famine, claim that it was the fundamental failure of the government to respond to the changing circumstances that lay at the heart of the crisis.[40] They point out that the strategy of the North Korean government in continuing to suppress private production and trade in grain, and monopolizing distribution through the Public Distribution System instead of introducing reforms, aggravated the food shortage. South Korean economic historian Suk Lee disagrees. Based on a meticulous assessment of a wide range of sources, including officially released North Korean statistics, Lee asserts that no feasible policies could have prevented the famine. He argues that a relatively low level of demographic loss was achieved due to the systematic coping strategies developed by the North Korean government to alleviate the famine.[41]

These differences in interpretation notwithstanding, most analysts underline the fact that the roots of the severe food problems that North Korea experienced during the 1990s did not develop overnight; they lie in the very nature of its political and economic system. The failure in the long-term management of North Korean agriculture is considered the most important component of the disaster. As it evolved from private farming to cooperative farming under local planning (1953–73) and then centralized planning (1973–87), the North Korean agricultural system became increasingly vulnerable.

After the swift implementation of land reform in 1946 (see chapter Four), the next stage in reforming North Korean agriculture was collectivization. The formation of state farms from confiscated land reserved as state property was in the first place intended to demonstrate the superiority of collective management of the rural economy. Soon, however, these farms began to function as the forerunners for cooperativization en masse, with the labour shortage caused by the Korean War acting as a catalyst that speeded up the process. Various kinds of mutual aid groups that sprang up between 1950 and 1953 evolved into incipient forms of cooperatives with the support of the government. By the end of the war the number of cooperatives had reportedly reached 174, involving 2,354 households. In the following two years the state intensified the preferential treatment of cooperatives over individual farmers by reducing their taxes-in-kind, renting them machinery and giving them priority access to high-quality seed. This resulted in phenomenal growth by cooperatives, from 31.8 per cent of all peasant households at the end of 1954 to 49 per cent a year later, and 80.9 per cent in December 1956. By August 1958 the entire rural population of North Korea was under a cooperative management system.[42]

As cooperative farms became the basic production unit, farm operations from production to marketing came under direct state control, despite the fact that the farms were formally owned by member households rather than the government. However, during the first decade of its operation, the system was highly decentralized. The role of the Agricultural Commission (Nong'ŏp Wiwŏnhoe) – the agricultural ministry in Pyongyang – was confined to providing advice on long-term agricultural development. Two of the most important policy decisions of the early 1960s were the identification of regional self-sufficiency as the guiding principle of North Korean agriculture and the modernization programme that was to be achieved through mechanization, irrigation, electrification (indispensable for setting up complex irrigation systems) and chemicalization.[43] The two institutions that directly determined the operation of cooperative farms were the Provincial Rural Management Committee – a state agricultural agency that functioned like a central planner in each province – and the County Cooperative Management Commission (CCMC), a state agricultural agency that supervised the operation of cooperative farms in each county. The latter also owned all of the assets that were necessary for the farm to operate, including its water supply and farm equipment, and provided technological support in the form of technicians and agricultural specialists.[44]

The average North Korean cooperative farm (*hyŏptong nongjang*) consisted of roughly 300 households, 1,500 people and 500 *chŏngbo* of arable land.[45] It was run by a Management Committee, composed of between fifteen and twenty members, and supervised by its Auditing Committee, composed of between five and fifteen members (see p. 185,

Chart v). Each farm usually had two production guidance workers who were engaged principally in administrative work, at least one agricultural specialist (usually a graduate of an agricultural college) who was responsible for the introduction of advanced technology, a planner-statistician, two to four bookkeepers, one or two labour statisticians and one or two warehouse custodians. Over 90 per cent of the total number of able-bodied members of the farm, both men and women over sixteen years of age, were organized into two main 'work teams' (*chagŏppan*): *nongsan chagŏppan* (the 'agricultural production work team') and *ch'uksan chagŏppan* (the 'animal husbandry work team'), plus smaller teams specializing in growing fruit and vegetables, sericulture and so on. Each work team was divided into 'work sub-teams' (*punjo*) with between two and twenty members depending on the type of activity. In other words, in a cooperative farm the household was no longer a unit of production, and independent peasants became rural proletarian workers.[46]

The primary motivation behind the shift to cooperative farming during the 1950s was a strong conviction that the goal of national self-sufficiency in terms of food production could not be achieved by the small-scale private farming system ruined by the Korean War, especially given the post-war shortage of resources.[47] This principle has guided the agricultural policies of the North Korean regime from the very beginning, in accord with the principle of 'self-reliance economy' (*chuch'e kyŏngje*). *Chuch'e* (literally 'self-reliance'), better known as the incorrectly romanized '*juche*', is the doctrine of self-reliance and independence, which since the mid-1950s developed as the state ideology of North Korea. The doctrine evolved around two concepts: 1) that man is the master of his destiny (and he should achieve this by subordination to the leader); and 2) that he should never become spiritually or psychologically dependent on outside assistance.[48] Ironically, while pursuing the goal of a self-sufficient food supply, the North Korean government became increasingly dependent on imported fertilizers and machinery (see below).

As explained above, during the first decade of cooperative farming the system was highly decentralized. However, in response to grain production failures between 1970 and 1973, which were caused by a combination of bad weather and insufficient input of resources, Kim Il-sung (1912–1994) personally intervened in agricultural practices, ordering an immediate shift from local to centralized planning. This shift away from the principle of independent local management of agriculture in each province was achieved not by restructuring the existing system, but by the agricultural ministry in Pyongyang assuming direct control over local institutions. Since no institutional channels existed to influence agricultural planning and resource allocation in each province, this was achieved through a series of directives, later grouped under the name *chuch'e nongpŏp* (literally 'self-reliance farming method'). The directives standardized all agriculture-related decisions and practices. For example, they defined precisely how widely, deeply and evenly a labourer should plough the field and what the ratio between fertilizer consumption and agricultural output should be. They specified how many tractors and labourers should be mobilized to plough one hectare of land, how many labourers could substitute the work of one tractor and so forth. In practice, the 'self-reliance farming method', which in 1979 was declared the only farming method that could be practised in DPRK, deprived local administrators of their authority to conduct agricultural planning and resource allocation in each prefecture independently. Moreover, as Lee explains, 'because all detailed production processes in agriculture were standardised and forced by the government, farm households also completely lost their autonomy/influences in production. There was now no difference between simple industrial labourers and farm households in production.'[49]

This shift from decentralized agriculture managed by the authorities of each province to the centralized planning regulated by the central government proved successful at first sight, as grain production increased at an average of 4.62 per cent per annum between 1973 and 1987 (see p. 181, Table XII). The growth was pursued by intensifying the three-tiered strategy of North Korean agriculture that had been introduced earlier: 1) a persistent increase in grain-sown area; 2) a continuous shift from low-yield to high-yield grains (in particular rice and maize); and 3) maximizing agricultural input through irrigation, chemicalization, mechanization and electrification. These three policies were responsible for a continuous growth in grain production in North Korea, from 1.9 million tonnes in 1946 to 10 million in 1987.[50]

Despite the seeming success of the measures introduced, in the long run these very same strategies ruined North Korean agriculture, and were indirectly responsible for the famine of the 1990s. Measures to expand arable land caused deforestation, which in turn reduced natural resistance against floods and droughts. As food-grain production was expanded to colder and more mountainous areas, it became increasingly vulnerable to weather conditions. Mono-cropping of rice and maize caused soil exhaustion, and the extensive use of fertilizers further damaged farmland conditions. In only twenty years, between 1949 and 1969, the average use of fertilizer per *chŏngbo* (approx. 0.99 hectares) increased from 131 to 500 kg.[51] A growing reliance on machinery and chemicals – in large part imported from the Soviet bloc – also made North Korean agriculture vulnerable to industrial stagnation and political tensions. In short, the North Korean agricultural system, as it kept evolving after the 1950s, grew increasingly vulnerable to external shocks.[52] Even the intervention of *chuch'e nongpŏp* failed to overcome the problems that, as underlined above, lay in the very nature of the North Korean agricultural system. The break-up of the USSR and the industrial collapse of North Korea were the last straws that set the system on the road to disaster. Between 1987 and 1996 grain production declined from 10 to 2.5 million tonnes according to the official North Korean statistics, and from 7.6 to 2.6 million according to FAO (UN Food and Agriculture Organization) data.[53]

The Public Distribution System (PDS) and Beyond

Unlike the chaotic condition of grain collection and distribution in the American occupation zone during the mid-1940s (see chapter Four), food rationing north of the 38th parallel continued more or less undisturbed, relying largely on the wartime organs of food management that had been instituted by the Japanese. Gradually, however, the system of state control of food evolved, adjusting to the unfolding political and economic changes. For example, by 1946 only the employees of state organs and state-run enterprises (roughly 18.6 per cent of the North Korean population) became entitled to food rations. In 1952 urban industrial cooperatives and private firms licensed by the government were also included in state food rationing, and six years later, when urban collectivization was completed, it was extended to all town dwellers (29.7 per cent of the population). With the collectivization of agriculture, which proceeded at approximately the same time, farmers (66.4 per cent of the population) also became recipients of state food rations.

Before collectivization, individual North Korean farmers remained independent and sustained themselves on their own produce. They were allowed, after delivery of 'agricultural tax-in-kind' to the authorities, to exchange any surplus grain for goods via consumer cooperatives or trade it at farmers' markets (*nongmin sijang*). Markets were held in every city and county ranging from daily to biweekly, with prices regulated by local 'price control committees'. Nearly 500 markets were in operation throughout North Korea in 1948, and by 1950 'market management stations' were in place, entrusted with collecting market fees, monitoring trade items and prices, and maintaining security and order.[54] The mass rural collectivization completed in the late 1950s put an end to the entrepreneurship of the farmer and private trade in grain. All grain markets were banned in 1958 and 'tax-in-kind' abolished in 1966.[55] Cooperative farms were required to turn all their produce over to the state and each farm worker received his or her ration from the cooperative.

Following the Japanese template, the quantities of a standard grain ration to be distributed varied depending on gender, age and type of employment (see p. 181, Table XIII). Officially, the categories and quantities of grain ration remained unchanged until 1972. However, there were temporary (unofficial) reductions at times of crisis. For example, some time around 1968–9 the government reduced rations by 3 kg per person per month (equal to four days' rations).[56] Official cuts began in 1973 with the so-called 'wartime grain reserves' reduction of approximately 13 per cent, followed by a further 10 per cent 'patriotic grain' reduction in 1987, and yet another adult reduction of 10 per cent (except for the army and heavy indistry workers) five years later.[57] Afterwards, the actual distribution never matched the norm nationwide and the PDS system nearly collapsed in the mid-1990s. Moreover, due to the principle of regional self-sufficiency in food supply, great regional differences emerged in the actual quantities of grain rationed to non-farming consumers. For example, in 1998 the annual PDS ration per capita in Kangwŏn was a mere 21 kg, nearly half of the 41 kg distributed in Pyongyang. Those who received rations in South Hamgyŏng Province and North Hamgyŏng Province, where the first wave of starvation emerged in 1994, were issued 25 and 28 kg respectively, while recipients in the city of Kaesŏng received 31 kg, Ryanggang 35 kg and Chagang 40 kg.[58]

In principle, farm rations corresponded to the rations for workers in heavy industry (800 grams of grain per day). However, farmers received their annual rations in advance shortly after the harvest, before the grain was handed over to the authorities for distribution among non-farming households. The latter collected their rations every fifteen days through the Public Distribution System, a permanent institution of the Democratic People's Republic of Korea that has officially continued to supply staple foods to the North Korean population until the present day.[59] This difference in issuing procedure explains the urban character of the 1990s famine: while farmers secured their share before the grain collection, the non-farming population – 60 per cent of the population of North Korea in 1993 – had to make do with what was left. Since the central government shifted grain deliveries between different areas to alleviate food shortages, urban communities were not infrequently left with no food for prolonged periods of time.

Moreover, farmers were permitted to retain a small plot of land – officially not larger than 160 square metres – to be used for growing vegetables and fruit, and for the small-scale raising of livestock for their own consumption and trade at farmers' markets. These plots not only placed farmers in an advantageous position in terms of food supply, but also constituted the very seed of the revival of a market economy in the late 1990s and early 2000s. As farmers increasingly concentrated on farming private plots to supplement the deficits, the markets gradually transformed into trade hubs.[60]

From the very beginning of the North Korean food rationing system allocations differed not only in the amount of food, but also in its quality, with higher-grade rations including higher proportions of white rice.[61] Generally speaking, during the 1960s, when the economic situation in North Korea was relatively sound, rice comprised 70–80 per cent of the grain ration. By the 1970s, however, rice constituted the bulk of the grain ration only in Pyongyang, while the rest of the population had to rely primarily on barley and maize.[62] The military and the party elite were the exception and received their rations primarily in rice. They remained privileged even at the eve of the famine, as Table XIII reveals. The first three groups represented the so-called 'centrally supplied population', which not only retained the right to be supplied primarily with rice while their countrymen were on the verge of starvation, but also used different distribution channels from the 'generally supplied population'.

The grain ration for non-farmers could be collected at distribution centres in each neighbourhood (*tong*). Shops were administered by the government administrative committee in each neighbourhood, serving approximately 1,000–1,200 families. The residents were expected to shop in their own neighbourhood stores; food rations could not be redeemed elsewhere.[63] Among the accounts of North Korean defectors collected by Barbara Demick is a detailed description of ration collection by the aforementioned Mrs Song:

> For as long as she was married, Mrs Song had gone every fifteen days with two plastic shopping bags to the same food distribution center. It was right in the neighborhood, tucked between two apartment complexes. This wasn't like a supermarket where you plucked what you wanted from the shelf; the women waited in line outside an unmarked storefront with a big metal gate that swung open. Everybody had their assigned days – Mrs Song's were the third and the eighteenth – but still there was often a wait of several hours. Inside there was a small, unheated room with white concrete walls, and a cheerless woman sitting behind a small table covered with ledger books. Mrs Song would hand over her ration book, a small sum of money, and coupons from the garment factory certifying that she had fulfilled her work duty. The clerks would calculate her entitlements: 700 grams each per day for her and Chang-bo; another 300 grams for her mother-in-law, since retired people got less; and 400 for each child still living at home. If anybody in the family was travelling, the rations for the days out of town would be deducted. Once the calculations were made, the clerk would pick up the official seal and with a self-important thump pound it into the red ink and onto receipts in triplicate, one of which she'd give to Mrs Song. At the back of the warehouse, where they stored big vats of rice, corn, barley, and flour, another clerk would weigh out the rations and put them into Mrs Song's plastic bags.[64]

Supplementary food items such as vegetables, soybean paste, salt, cooking oil and sugar entered the rationing system as well, starting in borderland cities in 1967 and followed by Pyongyang three years later. By the 1980s, as Andrei Lankov reports in his collection of essays on daily life in the northern half of the Korean peninsula, nothing could be bought freely in North Korean stores, which were virtually turned into distribution centres.[65] As was the case with the grain ration, only inhabitants of a particular neighbourhood could buy food at the neighbourhood's shop using food coupons. The sale of vegetables in bulk was also practised. For example, trucks delivered cabbage for winter *kimch'i* to each neighbourhood, where every family, regardless of the number of persons, was entitled to the same quantity.[66]

Different kinds of food coupons were in circulation in North Korea. Rationing coupons (*singnyang-gwŏn/-p'yo*) were issued by the payroll office of the state and distributed by the employer. Retired individuals received their coupons through their neighbourhood 'people's groups' (*inminban*) – North Korean successors of the wartime 'patriotic units' (see chapter Four) – and students through their schools.[67] Additional 'purchasing coupons' (*kumaegwŏn*) and 'goods allocation coupons' (*sangp'um paejŏngp'yo*) were usually distributed through employers. Rationing coupons were required also when one ate away from home, in a company's cafeteria or hospital, although some large factories did provide additional meal services to their employees. Special travel food coupons (*kich'apap p'yo*) could also be redeemed, but needed to be applied for in advance.[68]

State enterprises that employed the non-farming population were also involved in supplying their workers with food by following three strategies. First of all, state enterprises could purchase surplus foodstuffs directly from cooperative farms and distribute them among their employees. While cooperative farms were required to turn in their entire grain production and industrial crops to the authorities, they were allowed – and after 1987 even encouraged – to sell surplus vegetables, fruit and livestock (after fulfilling delivery quotas) to state enterprises or directly to consumers at farmers' markets.[69] As a second option, enterprises could operate food production facilities, such as livestock farms and kitchen gardens, and allocate industrial workers farming hours to work in those facilities. This option came to be known as the Daean Work System, from the Daean Electric Factory, which came up with the idea. In essence, Daean Factory operated its own food production facilities to feed its 5,000 employees: 70 *chŏngbo* of land for vegetables, another 80 for fruit, a chicken farm producing 45,000 eggs per day and a pig farm on a similar scale.[70]

Finally, an enterprise could assign plots for kitchen gardens and farming hours to their employees, who could cultivate them individually. This strategy was encouraged by the authorities at the time when they introduced a 10 per cent cut in grain rations in 1987.[71] At the same time, farmers were permitted to expand their private plots and, more importantly, for the first time in decades the tilling of grain on those plots and trading it at farmers' markets was tolerated. By 1995 all regulations concerning private plots of farm households and sales of this produce had been lifted altogether.[72] The liberalization of private farming and the food trade was the first indicator that the crumbling

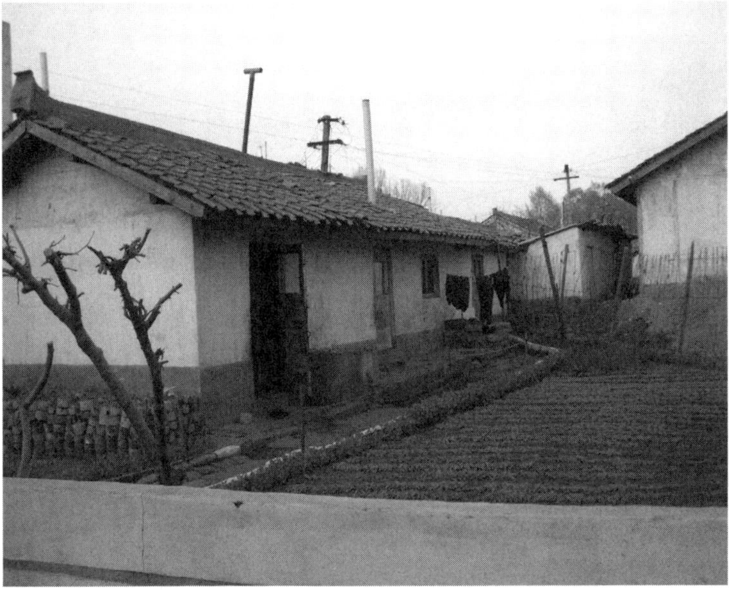

A North Korean kitchen garden, 2008.

of the North Korean agricultural system would eventually lead to the expansion, however modest, of the market economy. Reports by defectors indicated that an average farmer could produce as much as 200 kg of grain on his private plot by spending two to three days cultivating it, while he received 180 kg of grain from the cooperative farm for 256 days of work.[73]

Already in 1984 new regulations extended the operation of farmers' markets, allowing private trade on a daily basis. Before the 1990s the range of goods on sale was small, including apples, homemade sweets, ducks, chickens, fish and potatoes. No staple foods – rice or other grains – were to be traded at those markets.[74] Still, they formed the seed of the explosion in private trade that took place during the 1990s, transforming the markets from 'farmers' markets' (*nongmin sijang*) into 'open-air markets' (*changmadang*). According to the report by the ROK Ministry of Unification, roughly 300–350 officially recognized markets were in operation throughout the country in 1998, on top of many railway stations that functioned as unrecognized markets.[75] In recent years private food stalls have begun to pop up outside the markets as well.[76] The relaxation of restrictions on domestic travel also provided an important stimulus for private trade to thrive.

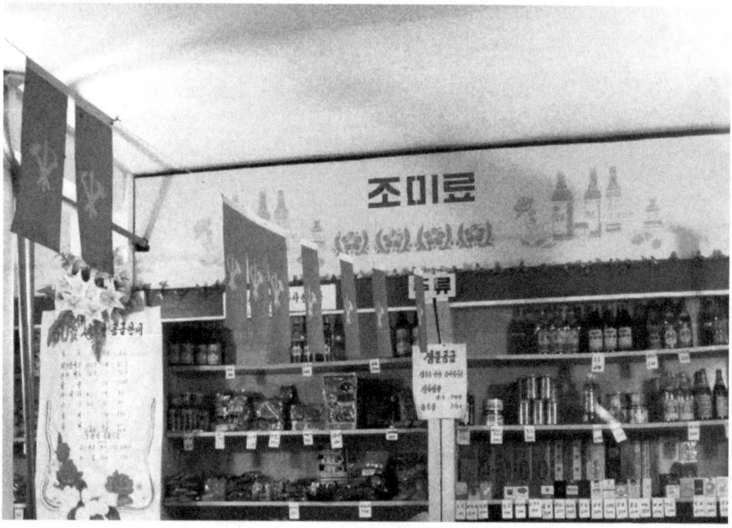

A grocery shop in Pyongyang, 2005.

Private markets have become the centres of North Korean economic life and for many the lifeline through which to escape starvation. In 1999 the average North Korean acquired an estimated 60 per cent of his or her food supply through those markets. While the markets remained largely under government control (with upper price limits set by the authorities), the goods were affordable only for those who managed to secure other sources of income apart from their state salary. For example, in the mid-1990s, 1 kg of pork cost 20 won – one-third of an average monthly salary – and the price of a chicken was 40 won.[77] An FAO/WFP report compiled on a visit in 2008 to Tong-il market, one of the official markets around Pyongyang, confirmed that food prices were five to ten times higher than at state shops.

> A wide range of food commodities from vegetables, to fruit, fish and meat were being sold in well setup concrete stalls/tables. Each commodity group had its own corner; for instance, the meat section had pork, dog meat, chicken and ducks in reasonably good quantities. The fish section had diverse types of fish of varying sizes.[78]

The days of the PDS being the sole source of nutrition for the urban population are definitely over. Although it recovered from a near-collapse in the mid-1990s, it remains highly unreliable. For example, in 2004–5 the daily ration issued was a mere 200–250 grams per person per day – less than the 2.3 *gō* (330 grams) wartime Japanese ration six decades earlier. By October 2005 the rations are reported to have increased to 500 grams per day, but were lowered again to 300–400 grams due to floods in August 2007. Moreover, rations tend to fluctuate by season, reaching a peak in November and December when new grains are collected. For example, the 350 grams issued at the beginning of 2008 were reduced to 250 grams in May and further to 150 grams between June and September before they were adjusted upwards to 300 grams in October.[79] Nonetheless, according to Suk Lee, it seems unlikely that the PDS will soon be abandoned as it constitutes a major mechanism of the DPRK government control over the urban population, which is vital for the regime's survival.[80]

Food and Eating in the Socialist Paradise

On 1 July 2002 the North Korean government devaluated the North Korean won against the United States dollar by 6,000–7,000 per cent, bringing food prices in North Korea closer to international levels. By dramatically raising retail prices, the state effectively got rid of the burden of subsidizing major foodstuffs that had for decades drained government finances. The price of rice increased by 55,000 per cent and the price of corn by 5,000 per cent, while wages rose on average by approximately 2,000 per cent.[81] Overnight the price of 1 kg of rice increased from 0.1 to 40 won, a hard reality for ordinary North Koreans with nothing to barter.

To be sure, North Korea has never been an egalitarian heaven with equal shares for everyone. Even before the famine a strong discrepancy persisted between the life of the elite and the remaining 90 per cent of the population. As under the Soviet system, the differences in the standard of living did not derive in North Korea from the differentiation of salaries or accumulation of wealth, but rather from access to a wide range of free benefits.[82] For example, while their salaries were modest (150–250 won per month), high-ranking officials could afford fine dining thanks to special monetary allowances. They resided in homes owned and furnished by the state, and were entitled to free issue of a wide range of goods. Elite cadres had access to stores with imported items and North Korean products reserved for export, such as beef,

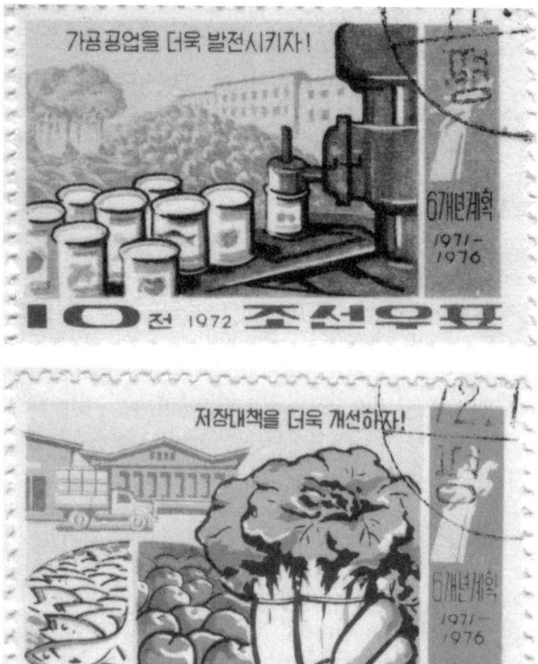

A set of North Korean stamps from 1972 promoting the '1971–1976 Six-year Plan', each with a different slogan: (top) 'Let's further develop the manufacturing process!'; (middle) 'Let's improve the storage policies!'; (bottom) 'Let's improve the packaging of products!'

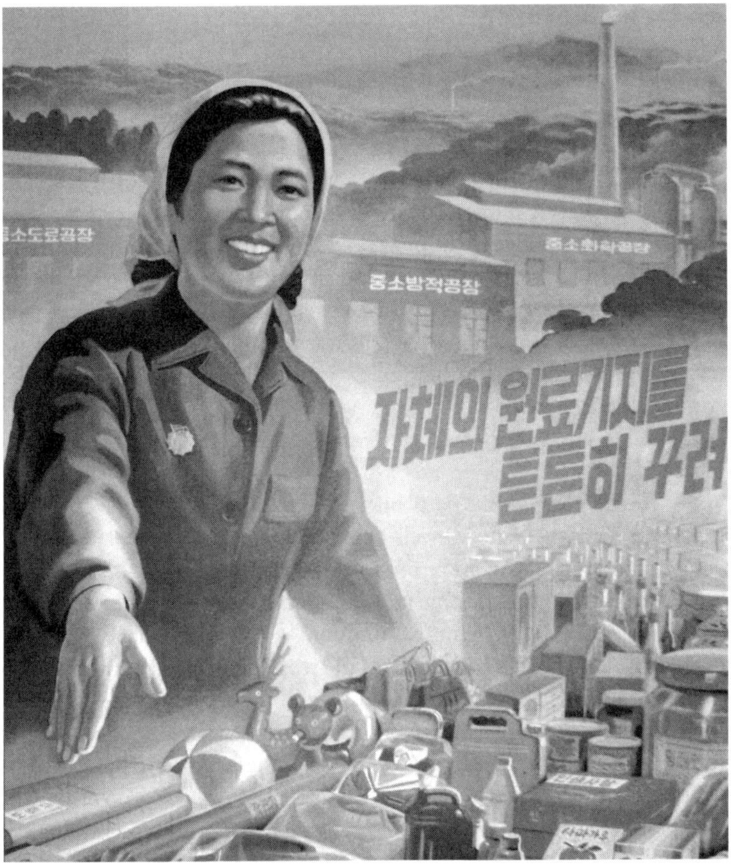

A North Korean propaganda poster with the slogan 'Let's increase the production of consumer goods!'

pork, eggs, fresh seafood, candy, wine and liquor. These commodities were rarely available outside these special stores even before the food crisis struck in the early 1990s.[83]

South Korean medical anthropologist Sunyoung Pak argues that although there were noticeable improvements in the infant mortality rate, maternal mortality rate, vaccination rate and medical facilities in North Korea between the 1940s and '70s, daily nutrition in the workers' paradise hardly changed over the decades. The minimal increase in the average height of the North Korean population indicates that increases in welfare have been quite modest or nonexistent.[84] Mean height is a recognized indicator of economic conditions in the long term.[85] The foundation of Pak's claim are the differences in heights of adults in North and South Korea, acquired through anthropometric studies conducted together with Daniel Schwekendiek among North Korean refugees who arrived in South Korea between 1999 and 2003 (2,384 adults between 20 and 70 years of age and 283 children and adolescents). Pak concluded that the mean height of North Koreans has only increased slightly during the course of the last 50 years. The increase among males is (at most) 0.8 cm, from 158 cm among those between 40 and 49 years old at the time of Pak's study (born in the 1950s) to 158.8 cm among those between 25 and 29 years old (born in the 1970s). This change in height was minimal compared to the 3.8 cm increase in the mean height of South Korean men between the comparable age groups. The pattern among females was similar in the comparable age groups: 0.6 cm versus 2.6 cm in North and South Korea respectively.[86]

These outcomes are particularly disappointing when one considers that improving the material well-being of workers has been a consistent goal of the North Korean regime from its outset. In fact, Armstrong argues that the emphasis on material conditions is 'one of the most distinctively Korean elements of communism in North Korea'.[87] Visions of the absence of material worries in the workers' paradise feature prominently in North Korean propaganda, and regularly included food as the central theme of the message. Propaganda posters frequently depict food in abundance, usually at the very moment of being harvested or produced, but hardly ever actually being consumed.[88] The emphasis was placed on the promise of plenty brought about by technological advancement in the production and processing of food. For example, a 1950s poster depicts a female factory worker proudly displaying her industrially processed foodstuffs, accompanied by the slogan 'Ahead to realize and surpass the 1955 People's Economic Plan!' Nearly two decades later, on the occasion of the launch of the Six-year Plan 1971–1976, the messages were more concrete: 'Let's further develop the manufacturing process!', 'Let's improve the storage policies!', and 'Let's improve the packaging of products!' One of the main goals of the plan was to free women from housekeeping work by increasing production of home appliances and pre-cooked food.[89]

The North Korean food-processing industry includes factories manufacturing soy sauce, soybean paste and *kimch'i*, as well as canneries, noodle factories, oil processing factories and alcohol distilleries. Maize-processing factories were ubiquitous, maize being the second major grain crop next to rice. Along with corn oil and corn syrup, 'corn rice' (*okssal*) – maize and wheat flour mixed with water and pressed into rice grain shapes – was also manufactured for distribution as a staple food ration. The so-called 'meal factories' (*pap kongjang*) also operated in cities between the 1960s and the '80s. *Pap kongjang* can be described as large-scale catering factories which delivered cooked meals to canteens and private families.[90]

The question that still remains unanswered at the end of this chapter is what North Koreans actually ate during the last half-century. The culinary history of North Korea deserves more attention than it has received thus far, but the available information is very scarce and largely overshadowed by the recent famine. Moreover, there seems to be a considerable discrepancy between the 'official story' of the relatively comfortable lives of the elite and the daily existence of the majority of the population. High-ranking officials among North Korean defectors openly acknowledge that they have never experienced any hardships with regard to food, while their less privileged counterparts hailing from rural areas provide details about meals that qualify as famine relief foods, such as rice cooked with corn germ dregs, a by-product in corn oil manufacture used worldwide as animal fodder (*chigemi pap*), and noodles made from a mixture of corn and potato flour and ground tree bark (*honhap kuksu*). These staple foods were familiar to the population of rural North Korea during the 1970s and '80s, and were in fact modern versions of the dishes Korean farmers had subsisted on for centuries.[91]

A WFP report from 2008 claimed that North Korean meals typically consisted of rice or maize, vegetable soup and a side dish of *kimch'i*, usually supplemented with seaweed, wild vegetables and herbs. Cabbage and beans are the two prevailing vegetables, followed by spinach, aubergine, cucumber, pumpkin, garlic, radish, onion, chilli and tomato.[92] The data collected through interviews with North Korean defectors confirms that a comparable meal pattern was characteristic of the pre-1990s North Korean diet. Rice, maize flour, 'corn rice', wheat flour and wheat noodles seem to have been the prevalent staples among city-dwellers, but not much was served on the side. *Kimch'i* and soup are mentioned as the most prevalent side dishes, followed by bean curd, eggs and fish on special occasions.[93] Andrei Lankov reports, based on his own experience, that during the 1980s meals served in canteens of student dormitories consisted usually of rice or corn gruel and *kimch'i*, 'with meat or even fish almost unheard of'.[94] Helen-Louise Hunter, a veteran chief analyst of North Korea for the CIA who has conducted interviews with North Korean defectors since the 1970s, reports that meat at subsidized prices used to be rationed to North Korean households on the five national holidays: New Year's Day, Kim Il-sung's birthday (15 April), May Day, Liberation Day (15 August) and National Founding Day (9 September), and that the consumption of meat among the ordinary population was restricted to these occasions.[95] Meat was consumed only sporadically in South Korea, too, before economic affluence transformed it from a luxury to a fixture of the daily diet (see chapter Five). A survey of rural villages conducted in South Korea between 1972 and 1974 revealed that 80–90 per cent of calories consumed by farmers came from carbohydrates, primarily grain.[96] In this respect the North Korean diet embodies (South) Korea's past before it fell victim to self-indulgence, consumerism and global culinary trends.

Conclusion

Due to its intricate connection with human nourishment and comfort, food stands as central to the life of every individual. Owing to its connection with profit and power, it also plays a critical role in the social and economic organization of societies.[1] What we eat, how we produce and distribute our food, who prepares it and how we think about it – as traditional or modern, local or national, 'foreign' or not, and most importantly tasty or not – are in a constant state of flux, continuously affected by the flow of history. Thus what happens to food and eating reflects on a micro level the consequences of macro-level political and economic processes. The ubiquitous presence of food makes it a potent signifier of the ordinary, disclosing history in its rawest form. As elsewhere, the culinary culture of contemporary Korea is a product of its past, and traces of the past are revealed in the diet of the Korean people. This book is an attempt to bring to light the raw history of modern Korea as it has been digested through the turbulent decades of the twentieth century.

The food odyssey of twentieth-century Korea described here begins with the colony as a breadbasket of the Japanese empire. While the production and processing of the fruits of Korean agriculture, animal husbandry and fisheries were subordinated to the goals of the colonizer, the consumption practices that emerged in the colonial cities were conceived in the context of the Japanese as trendsetters. Japanese urban culture was transplanted into Korea and the latest Western fashions were usually adopted through the Japanese filter.

As a growing body of evidence indicates, Japanese colonial domination had a critical impact on a wide range of economic, social and cultural transformations that took place in Korea during the first half of the twentieth century. Moreover, the colonial legacy continued

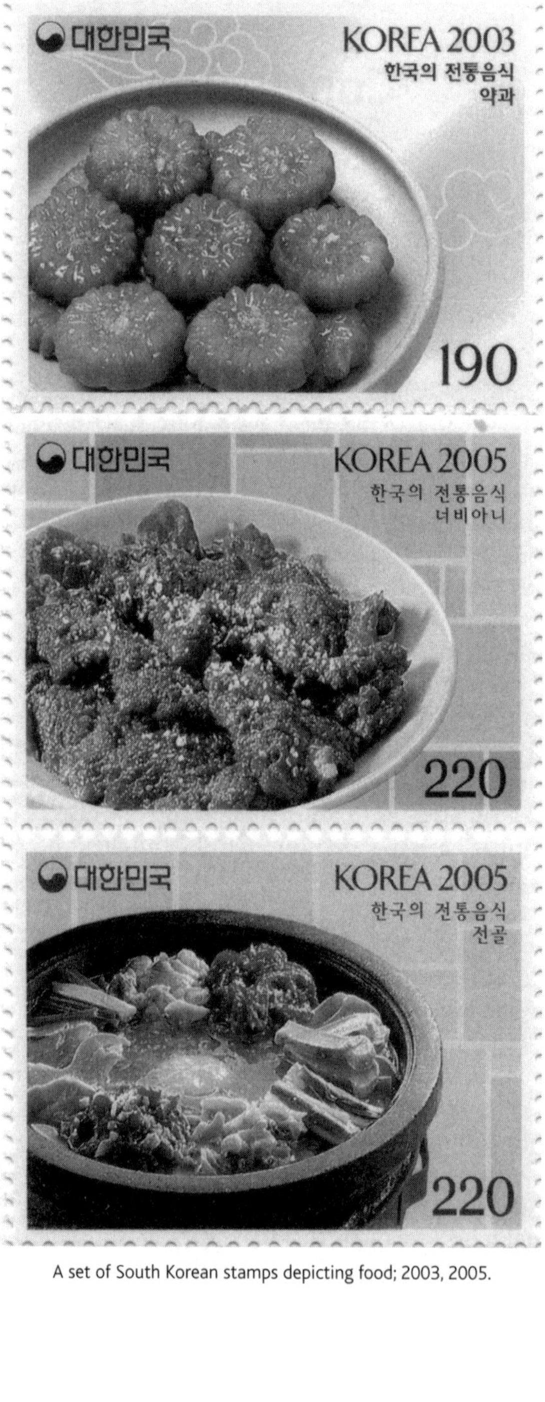

A set of South Korean stamps depicting food; 2003, 2005.

to impinge on Korea after 1945, and remains a contentious issue until the present day. One of the objectives of this volume has been to highlight the colonial and postcolonial connections in the dietary context. Such continuities have already been identified by political and economic historians,[2] but are more difficult to pin down in terms of the mundane reality of the everyday, which tends to be much less systematically documented.

It was the intensifying of Japanese militarist ambitions during the 1930s, along with the mid-twentieth century waging of war, that seems to have left the strongest and longest lasting imprint on food and eating on the Korean peninsula. The wartime system of state food management created by the colonizer under the pressure of the Sino-Japanese War and Pacific War to deal with scarce resources remained in place long after Korea's liberation. This particular aspect of the colonial legacy set the stage for decades of state control over diet in postcolonial Korea, and the Korean War helped to distance the system from the stigma of association with Japanese colonialism. The militarized context of the Cold War was crucial in fortifying and adapting wartime colonial practices for the new purpose of an ideological struggle between North and South. In other words, it was war – both 'hot' and 'cold' – that strengthened the dietary legacy of Japanese colonial rule on the Korean peninsula.

While facilitating continuity in terms of food distribution, mid-twentieth-century war-waging in Korea also inflamed dietary change. While the Korean population was deprived of its rice, seafood and beef in order to sustain the Japanese troops, Japanese facilities and production know-how in soy sauce and beer set the stage for the diffusion of these products in postcolonial Korea. On the other hand, the decades of American presence in the south were instrumental in inculcating among South Korean citizens the taste for luncheon meat, candy and other components of the U.S. Army ration, in the long run making the country dependent on American food imports. Sidney Mintz's claim that 'war is probably the single most powerful instrument of dietary change in human experience' fits perfectly in the South Korean context, especially if one considers that participation in the Vietnam War largely sustained the economic growth and culture of consumption that South Koreans are able to enjoy today.[3]

The recent outburst of appreciation for the Korean culinary heritage in South Korea and the increasing investment in promoting Korean culinary tradition as a globally recognizable commodity reflects

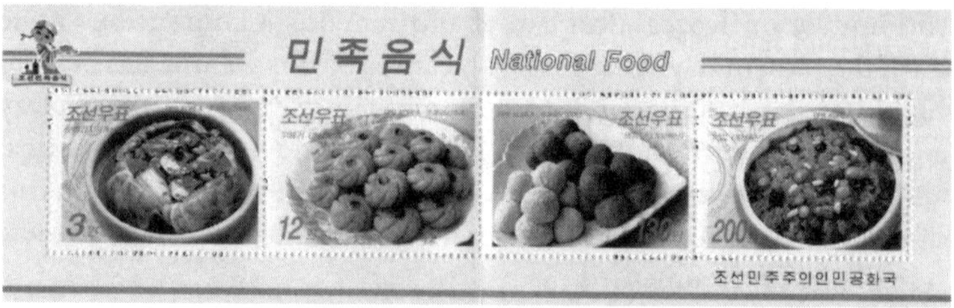

A set of North Korean stamps on the theme 'National Food', 2006.

the magnitude of the changes in the South Korean daily diet since the 1980s. An important implication of these changes is the growing divide between the consumption patterns of South Koreans and their Northern neighbours. While urbanization and economic affluence turned most South Koreans into sterile consumers, detached from any connection with the production and processing of food, the North Korean food shortages transformed masses of North Koreans into farmers and food vendors. While culinary nostalgia inspires South Koreans to embrace the half-invented traditions of the past, the majority of North Koreans are compelled to rely on the famine relief remedies of their ancestors.

Since Korea's liberation and the Korean War that followed, Koreans have been a 'divided' nation. Although the peninsula has officially been at war for over half a century, a fantasy that the division of the nation – which has disrupted Korean cultural and national identity and homogeneity – will some day be recovered through unification is widely diffused among South Koreans. The tension between the unified nation as an idealized past and future, and the divided nation as the world in which nearly every South Korean has been born and raised, is one of the most powerful components of South Korean identity.[4] South Korea has become a nation in which nearly all aspects of economic, political and cultural identity are defined in opposition to the North; a nation in which the public consciousness is saturated with a variety of different kinds of representations of North Korea. They range from negative ones, depicting North Koreans as uncivilized, brainwashed and backward people, to positive, romanticized images of 'primordial Koreans before the fall of the south into the evils of modernity', preserving traditions that the South Koreans have forgotten.[5]

North Korea as the romanticized cradle of Korean culinary tradition plays an important role in the positive image of North Korea in the South. Since the historic summit meeting in 2000, when the South

Korean president Kim Dae-jung (1925–2003) flew to Pyongyang to meet the North Korean leader Kim Jong-il (1942–2011), the image of North Korea as the 'nostalgic past', good old Korea frozen in time, has grown into a powerful marketing tool for North Korean products. Despite the end of the so-called Sunshine Policy – a South Korean policy of peaceful co-existence and economic cooperation with the North launched by President Kim Dae-jung – South Korean fantasies of finding their lost former selves in the economically deprived North trigger interest in North Korean food.[6]

The South Korean nostalgic longing for an ideal, aestheticized rural past is, unusually, saturated with the perception of suffering, since this past has not so much been 'lost' in Korea, but taken away by someone else.[7] The turbulent twentieth century has brought suffering to the Korean people, and despite their recently achieved affluence South Koreans see themselves foremost as the victims of history. The Japanese colonial exploitation occupies a prominent place in the public memory of twentieth-century dietary deprivation, rather than the corruption and authoritarian policies of postcolonial regimes. Even more than hunger and suffering, a striking continuity in Korea's twentieth-century odyssey depicted from the perspective of food is revealed in the exceptional longevity of state involvement in the matter of food and eating – a grip that began with the Japanese colonization, was tightened by mid-twentieth-century war-waging and the Cold War, and continues until the present day, in the North through the Public Distribution System and in the South via more subtle means.

The campaign to promote Korean cuisine abroad, instigated by the South Korean government in 2009, has multilayered implications that belie the seemingly trivial nature of the initiative. Elevating Korean culture to global supremacy is not the only issue at stake. The inclusion of *naengmyŏn* (cold noodles) – the most famous dish of the North – in the pantheon of Korean food as reinvented by South Korean spin doctors for global consumption invites a polemic on who owns the property rights to North Korean food. The images of Korean food distributed by the North Korean government strikingly resemble those issued by the South Korean post office. Where, then, lies the legitimate source of the authentic Korean culinary tradition?

Tables and Charts

Tables

I: Population of Korea, 1900–44[1]

Year	Koreans	Japanese	Japanese as % of Total
1900	12,000,000*	15,829	0.1
1910	14,766,000	171,543	1.3
1920	17,764,000	347,900	2.0
1930	20,438,000	501,900	2.5
1940	24,326,300	712,583	2.9
1944	25,133,352	752,830**	3.0

* estimated ** record as of 1942

II: Restaurants, tea rooms and cafés advertised in a tourist booklet, 1934[2]

NAME	LOCATION
Japanese Cuisine	
Sakuragi	Asahimachi, block 1
Chiyoshin	Asahimachi, block 1
Hakusui	Asahimachi, block 1
Kagetsu Villa	Nanzanchō, block 2
Kyōgiku	Asahimachi, block 2
Kiragu	Nanzanchō, block 2
Kishi no ryō	Asahimachi, block 2
Nanzansō	Nishi-shikenmachi
Hakuunsō	Seiunchō
Kamogawa sansō	Nanzanchō, block 2
Chiyomoto	Asahimachi, block 1
Kikuya	Honmachi, block 2
Miyakodori	Asahimachi, block 1
Kyōwatei	Asahimachi, block 1
Kagetsu main store	Honmachi, block 2

Korean Cuisine	
Meigetsukan main store (Myŏngwŏlgwan)	Tsūgimachi
Tenkōen (Ch'ŏnhyangwŏn)	Ninjichō

Cafeterias	
Kagetsu cafeteria (Japanese food)	Koganemachi
Keijō Station cafeteria	Keijō Station, first floor
Kagetsu cafeteria branch (Western food)	Hasegawachō
Chiyoda Grill	Chiyoda Bldg, Nandaimon Avenue

Cafés	
Marubiru Kaikan	Meijimachi
Salon Arirang	Arirang Ridge
Café Hikari	Honmachi, block 2
Kikusui	Koganemachi, block 2

Tea Rooms	
Meiji Confectionery Keijō store	Honmachi, block 2
Kameya Kongōsan tea room	Honmachi, block 2
Keijō Station tea room	Keijō Station

III: Number of soy sauce factories in each province, 1942–3[3]

Province	1941	1942
Kyŏnggi	40	46
N. Ch'ungch'ŏng	4	4
S. Ch'ungch'ŏng	13	13
N. Chŏlla	13	15
S. Chŏlla	15	17
N. Kyŏngsang	18	21
S. Kyŏngsang	47	53
Hwanghae	14	17
S. P'yŏngan	10	16
N. P'yŏngan	8	9
S. Hamgyŏng	14	18
N. Hamgyŏng	28	31
Kangwŏn	12	16

iv: Soy sauce factories in South Korea, 1963 and 1942[4]

Province	1963	1942
Kyŏnggi	44	46
N. Ch'ungch'ŏng	4	4
S. Ch'ungch'ŏng	12	13
N. Chŏlla	6	15
S. Chŏlla	7	17
N. Kyŏngsang	9	21
S. Kyŏngsang	38	53
Kangwŏn	9	16
Chaeju	2	?

v: Household staple food ration allowances for the non-farming population, as of May 1943[5]

Age Category	Allowance in Grams Per Day
1–2	120
3–5	120
6–10	250
11–15	360
16–60	330
Over 60	300
Pregnant women	350

vi: Price index of foodstuffs on the black market in Seoul, June 1944 (based on the assumption that the official price was equal to 1)[6]

Foodstuff	Price Index for Black Market
White rice	12 times higher
Small beans	11 times higher
Sesame seeds	15 times higher
Sweet potatoes	5 times higher
White potatoes	5.5 times higher
Apples	8 times higher
Beef	3.5 times higher
Pork	3.3 times higher
Eggs	4 times higher

Dried pollack	4.5 times higher
Sugar	10.5 times higher
Rice wine (*chŏngju*)	4 times higher
Rice cake	10 times higher

VII: Rationing of staple foods in North Korea, 1946–54[7]

Decree Issued	Recipient	Daily Ration Per Category
27/02/1946	Labourer, office worker and their dependants	Band 1: heavy labourer, 600 g Band 2: labourer, 500 g Band 3: office worker, 400 g Band 4: dependants, 300 g
19/10/1946	Labourer, office worker and their dependants	Special band: 900 g Band 1: heavy labourer, 750 g Band 2: labourer, 600 g Band 3: office worker and student, 525 g Band 4: dependants, 450 g
26/12/1946	Those who work in state organizations, state enterprises and private firms that the state regards as important, and their dependants	Band 1: heavy labourer, 700 g Band 2: labourer, 600 g Band 3: office worker, 500 g Band 4: dependants, 300 g
12/07/1947	Private firms are entitled to rations only for the period that they are directly involved in state economic planning	
27/03/1952	Those who work in the state sector, industrial collectives, private firms that the cabinet approves, and their dependants	Band 1: heavy labourer, 900 g Band 2: heavy labourer, 800 g Band 3: labourer, 700 g Band 4: office worker, 600 g Band 5: high school student, 500 g Band 6: primary school student, 400 g Band 7: infant in nursery, 300 g

VIII: Restaurants in Seoul according to the 'nationality' of served food, 1983–2003[8]

Year	Korean	Chinese	Japanese	Western	Total
1983	8,357	3,003	566	2,793	14,719
1993	26,909	3,994	2,293	9,586	42,782
2003	38,657	4,287	3,458	4,674	51,076

IX: Restaurants operating in South Korea according to the 'nationality' of served food, 1993–2006[9]

Year	Korean	Chinese	Japanese	Western
1993	151,438	19,379	5,331	12,696
2000	245,122	27,104	6,255	15,192
2003	277,136	25,080	5,067	13,991
2006	261,395	21,902	5,092	9,782

X: A typical weekly menu, side dishes to accompany rice, served by Ms Kim to her student boarders in September 2003 (in addition, two kinds of *kimch'i* and dried laver were served at every meal)[10]

DATE	SIDE DISHES SERVED
15/09	**Breakfast**: clear soup, simmered dried pollack, pieces of vegetables pan-fried in batter (*chŏn*), grilled fish. **Dinner**: *kimch'i* stew, simmered dried pollack, oyster *chŏtkal*, pieces of vegetables and fish pan-fried in batter, fried strips of devil's tongue (konjac) and fish cake.
16/09	**Breakfast**: seaweed (*miyŏk*) soup, sliced cucumber with hot sauce (*ch'ojang*) on the side, pieces of vegetables and fish pan-fried in batter, fried strips of devil's tongue and fish cake. **Dinner**: no record.
17/09	**Breakfast**: clear soup with bean sprouts, fried strips of devil's tongue and fish cake, sliced cucumber with hot sauce, shrimp *chŏtkal*, soybeans and dried baby sardines simmered in soy sauce, seasoned aubergine. **Dinner**: *kimch'i* stew, shrimp *chŏtkal*, soybeans and dried baby sardines simmered in soy sauce, stewed mackerel, seasoned aubergine, seasoned green-bean sprouts, small pieces of apple dressed in mayonnaise (referred to by Ms Kim as 'apple salad').

18/09 **Breakfast**: clear *kimch'i* soup with bean sprouts, the rest of side dishes exactly the same as the previous day's dinner.
Dinner: Dried pollack stew, shrimp *chŏtkal*, soybeans and dried baby sardines simmered in soy sauce, stewed mackerel, seasoned eggplant, seasoned green-bean sprouts, Ms Kim's 'apple salad', potatoes stewed with strips of fish cake, lightly pickled garlic stems (*changatchi*).

19/09 **Breakfast**: clear soup with bean sprouts, soybeans and dried baby sardines simmered in soy sauce, potatoes stewed with strips of fish cake, pickled garlic stems, sliced cucumber with hot sauce, spring onions and laver omelette, seasoned seaweed.
Dinner: no record.

20/09 **Breakfast**: clear soup with pollack, bean sprouts and egg, soybeans and dried baby sardines simmered in soy sauce, pickled garlic stems, seasoned courgette, sliced cucumber with hot sauce, fish and radish stew, fried egg (Western-style).
Dinner: clear soup with pollack, bean sprouts and egg, soybeans and dried baby sardines simmered in soy sauce, pickled garlic stem, sliced cucumber with hot sauce, seasoned courgette, fish and radish stew, stewed baby octopus.

21/09 **Breakfast**: clear soup with bean sprouts, soybeans and dried baby sardines simmered in soy sauce, pickled garlic stems, seasoned courgette, stewed baby octopus, boiled cabbage leaves and green peppers served with dipping sauce (*ssamjang*) on the side.
Dinner: clear soup with squid, soybeans and dried baby sardines simmered in soy sauce, pickled garlic stems, seasoned courgette, stewed baby octopus, cabbage leaves with dipping sauce.

XI: Production value of the South Korean food-processing industry, 1976 and 1986[11]

	1976	1986
Meat processing and preserving	143	3,009
Dairy products manufacturing	877	9,037
Fruit and vegetable processing	293	1,217
Marine products processing	886	8,799
Fats and oil processing	360	4,552
Cereals processing	2,273	5,284
Bread, cookie and noodle manufacturing	1,640	14,194
Sugar manufacturing	1,049	2,414

XII: Grain production and population growth in North Korea, according to the official DPRK statistics*[12]

	1946–73	1973–87	1987–97
Production growth	3.8%	4.62%	-12.32%
Population growth	3.2%	1.63%	1%

* although the levels of production in official statistics might be inflated, it is estimated that the increasing trend in grain production was real

XIII: Staple food rations in North Korea as of 1993, per employment group[13]

Group	Rice–Maize Ratio	Distribution	Amount
Members of the party politburo	100% rice or on demand	Every 2–3 days	700 g per day
Members of the party central committee, heads of departments in the party and Cabinet, party and government officials in Pyongyang and corresponding local officials	100% rice	Every 3–7 days or on demand	700 g per day
High-profile individuals in all social sectors	100% rice	Weekly or biweekly	700 g per day
Workers	Pyongyang: 60% rice Other Areas: 30% rice	Biweekly Biweekly	492 g per day 800 g per day
Industrial workers with heavy physical demands, such as miners	Pyongyang: 60% rice Other Areas: 30% rice	Biweekly	800 g per day
Farmers on state farms	Pyongyang: 60% rice Other Areas: 30% rice	Six months' ration supplied at once, another six months' ration supplied biweekly	800 g per day
Farmers on cooperative farms	Varied	Annual ration supplied at once	260 kg per year

Charts

I: Production of HVP liquid by Suzuki Chemical Company (in *koku*), 1937–45[14]

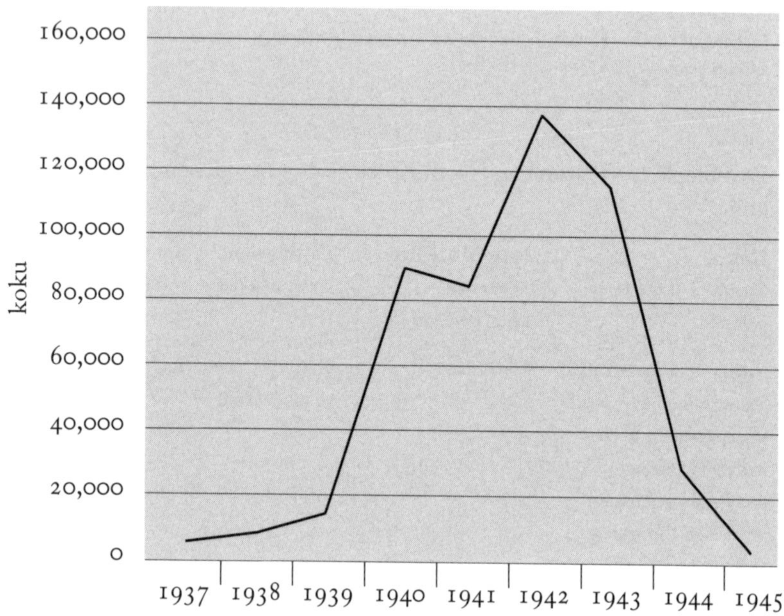

1 *koku* = approx. 180 litres

II: Average volume of production per factory in each province, 1942[15]

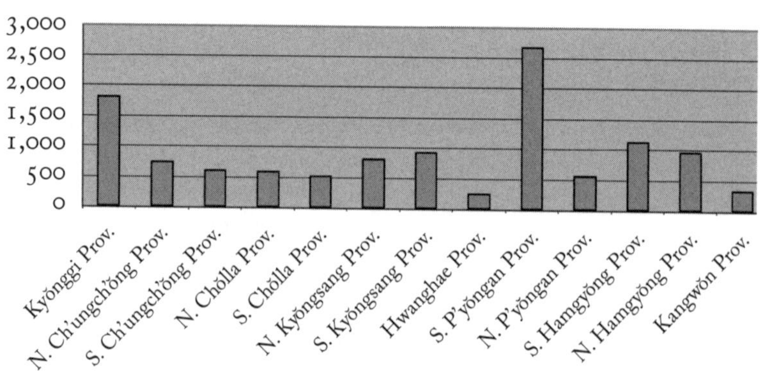

III: Korean rice exports to Japan, 1938–45 (in thousand tonnes)[16]

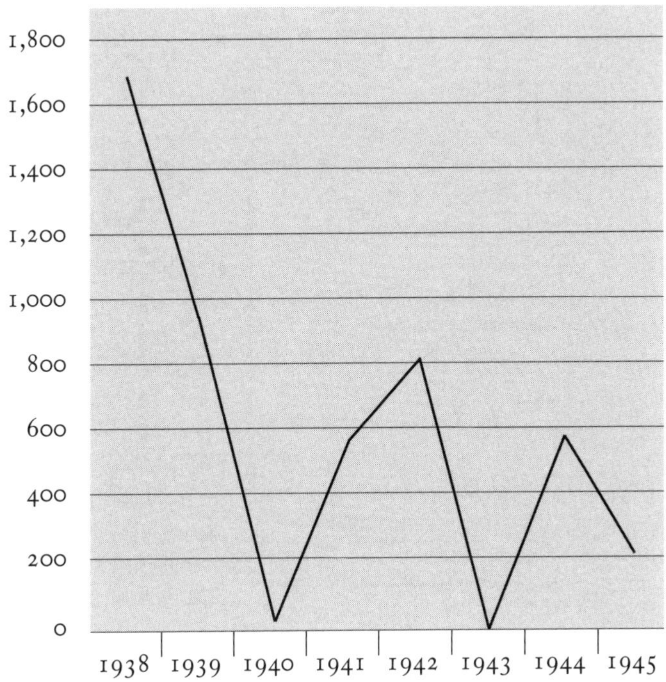

IV: Rough sketch of the meat rationing system of Keijō[17]

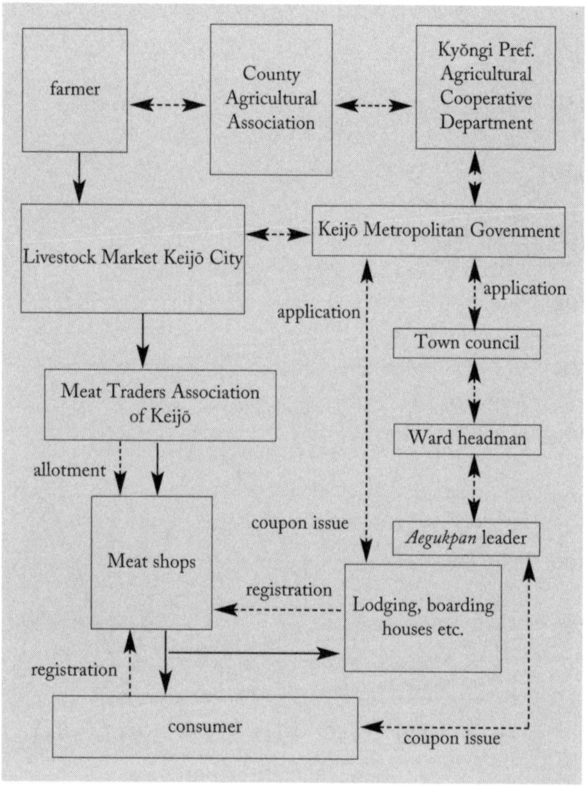

Solid lines indicate the flow of goods (meat) and dotted lines indicate the distribution of repsonsibilities

v: Cooperative farm organization[18]

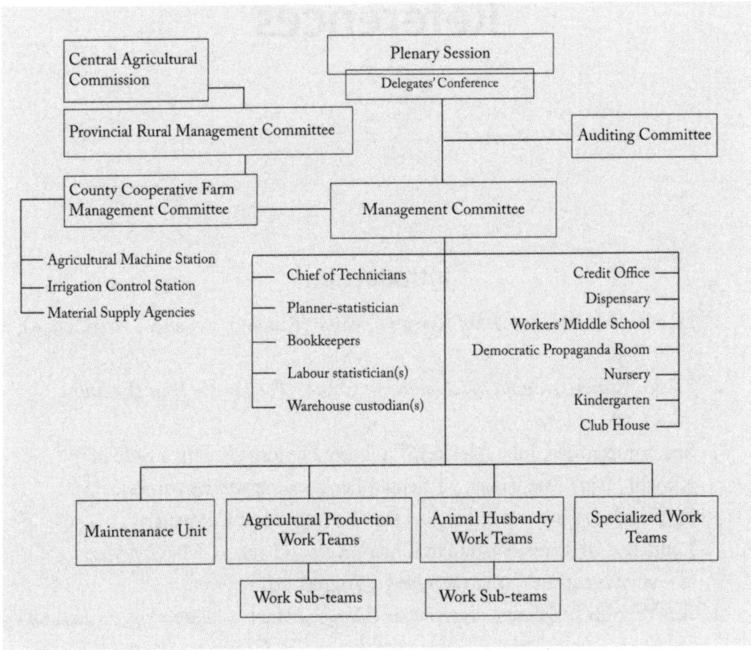

References

Introduction

1 Harriett Morris, *The Art of Korean Cooking* (Rutland, VT, and Tokyo, 1959), front flap.

2 J.A.G. Roberts, *China to Chinatown: Chinese Food in the West* (London, 2002), pp. 151–5.

3 See, for example, Julia Moskin, 'Culinary Diplomacy with a Side of Kimchi', *New York Times*, 22 September 2009, at www.nytimes.com (accessed 4 April 2012); Do Je-Hae, 'Korean Food Campaign Launched in Three Australian Cities', *Korea Times*, 25 March 2010, at www.koreatimes.co.kr (accessed 3 August 2011).

4 See Warren J. Belasco, *Appetite for Change: How the Counterculture Took on the Food Industry* (Ithaca, NY, 1989); Donna R. Gabaccia, *We Are What We Eat: Ethnic Food and the Making of Americans* (Cambridge, MA, 1998); Lisa Heldke, *Exotic Appetites: Ruminations of a Food Adventurer* (New York and London, 2003).

5 For a detailed description of the pre-modern history of Korean cuisine see Michael J. Pettid, *Korean Cuisine: An Illustrated History* (London, 2008).

6 Ibid., pp. 33–7. For accounts on the role of rice in the Korean diet and identity see Hanhee Hahm, 'Rice and Koreans: Three Identities and Meanings', *Korea Journal*, XLV/2 (2005), pp. 89–106; Michael Reinschmidt, 'Rice in South Korean Life: The Transformation of Agricultural Icons', in *The Art of Rice: Spirit and Sustenance in Asia*, ed. Roy W. Hamilton (Los Angeles, CA, 2003), pp. 509–25; and Kwang-ok Kim, 'Rice Cuisine and Cultural Practice in Contemporary Korean Dietary Life', *Korea Journal*, L/1 (2010), pp. 11–34.

7 Pettid, *Korean Cuisine*, pp. 25, 31, 59–61.

8 Boudewijn C. A. Walraven, 'Bardot Soup and Confucians' Meat: Food and Korean Identity in Global Context', in *Asian Food: The Global and the Local*, ed. K. J. Cwiertka with B.C.A. Walraven (Honolulu, HI, 2002), pp. 102–3.

9 Pettid, *Korean Cuisine*, p. 45.
10 Young-ha Chu, 'Origin and Change in *Kimch'i* Culture', *Korea Journal*, XXXV/2 (1995), pp. 18–29.
11 Michael E. Robinson, *Korea's Twentieth-Century Odyssey: A Short History* (Honolulu, HI, 2007), p. 1.

1 Breadbasket of the Japanese Empire

1 Rikki Kersten, 'Neo-nationalism and the "Liberal School of History"', *Japan Forum*, XI/2 (1999), pp. 191–203.
2 For example Kirk Y. K. Kim, 'The Impact of Japanese Colonial Development on the Korean Economy', *Korea Journal*, XVII/1 (1977), pp. 12–21; Toshiyuki Mizoguchi, 'Economic Growth of Korea under the Japanese Occupation: Background of Industrialization of Korea, 1911–1940', *Hitotsubashi Journal of Economics*, XX/1 (1979), pp. 1–19; Bruce Cumings, 'The Legacy of Japanese Colonialism in Korea', in *The Japanese Colonial Empire, 1895–1945*, ed. R. H. Myers and M. R. Peattie (Princeton, NJ, 1984), pp. 478–96; Dennis L. McNamara, *The Colonial Origins of Korean Enterprise, 1910–1945* (Cambridge, 1990); Gi-wook Shin and Michael Robinson, eds, *Colonial Modernity in Korea* (Cambridge, MA, 1999); Theodore Jun Yoo, *The Politics of Gender in Colonial Korea: Education, Labor, and Health, 1910–1945* (Berkeley, CA, 2008); Janice C. H. Kim, *To Live to Work: Factory Women in Colonial Korea, 1910–1945* (Stanford, CA, 2009); Jun Uchida, *Brokers of Empire: Japanese Settler Colonialism in Korea, 1876–1945* (Cambridge, MA, 2011).
3 Gi-wook Shin, *Ethnic Nationalism in Korea: Genealogy, Politics, and Legacy* (Stanford, CA, 2006), pp. 41–57.
4 Michael E. Robinson, *Korea's Twentieth-Century Odyssey: A Short History* (Honolulu, HI, 2007), p. 78.
5 Carter Eckert, *Offsprings of Empire: The Koch'ang Kims and the Colonial Origins of Korean Capitalism, 1876–1945* (Seattle, WA, 1991), p. 50.
6 Carter J. Eckert et al., *Korea Old and New: A History* (Seoul, 1990), pp. 257–8.
7 Samuel Pao-San Ho, 'Colonialism and Development: Korea, Taiwan and Kwantung', in *The Japanese Colonial Empire, 1895–1945*, ed. R. H. Myers and M. R. Peattie (Princeton, NJ, 1984), p. 361.
8 Ramon H. Myers and Saburō Yamada, 'Agricultural Development in the Empire', in *The Japanese Colonial Empire*, ed. Myers and Peattie, pp. 433–4.
9 Jung-en Woo, *Race to the Swift: State and Finance in Korean Industrialization*

(New York, 1991), pp. 35–8; Carter J. Eckert, 'Total War, Industrialization, and Social Change in Late Colonial Korea', in *The Japanese Wartime Empire, 1931–1945*, ed. P. Duus, R. H. Myers and M. R. Peattie (Princeton, NJ, 1996), pp. 3–14.

10 Katarzyna J. Cwiertka, *Modern Japanese Cuisine: Food, Power and National Identity* (London, 2006), pp. 61–5.

11 Michael A. Schneider, 'The Limits of Cultural Rule: Internationalism and Identity in Japanese Responses to Korean Rice', in *Colonial Modernity in Korea*, ed. G. W. Shin and M. Robinson (Cambridge, MA, 1999), p. 99.

12 Penelope Francks, 'Rice for the Masses: Food Policy and the Adoption of Imperial Self-sufficiency in Early Twentieth-century Japan', *Japan Forum*, xv/1 (2003), pp. 125–46.

13 Ibid., p. 128.

14 Paul H. Kratoska, 'Commercial Rice Cultivation and the Regional Economy of Southeastern Asia, 1850–1950', in *Food and Globalization: Consumption, Markets and Politics in the Modern World*, ed. A. Nützenadel and F. Trentmann (Oxford, 2008), p. 81.

15 Yunshik Chang, 'Colonization as Planned Change: The Korean Case', *Modern Asian Studies*, v/2 (1971), p. 171.

16 Ho, 'Colonialism and Development', p. 371. See also Bruce F. Johnston, *Japanese Food Management in World War II* (Stanford, CA, 1953), pp. 49–52.

17 Thierry Bonzon and Belinda Davis, 'Feeding the Cities', in *Capital Cities at War: Paris, London and Berlin, 1914–1919*, ed. J. Winter and J. L. Robert (Cambridge, 1997), pp. 305–41.

18 Lothar Burchardt, 'The Impact of the War Economy on the Civilian Population of Germany During the First and Second World War', in *The German Military in the Age of Total War*, ed. W. Deist (Oxford/New York, 1985), pp. 46–7.

19 Chang, 'Colonization as Planned Change', pp. 172–3.

20 Seung-nam Lee, 'Analytical Study of Influxes of Korean Rice and the Korean Rice Production Development Program: 1910–1939', *Hokkaidō Daigaku Nōkei Ronsō*, 40 (1984), p. 181.

21 Chang, 'Colonization as Planned Change', pp. 172–3.

22 Ho, 'Colonialism and Development', pp. 363–4.

23 Ibid., p. 379.

24 Schneider, 'The Limits of Cultural Rule', p. 126.

25 Johnston, *Japanese Food Management*, p. 54.

26 Yujiro Hayami and Vernon W Ruttan, 'Korean Rice, Taiwan Rice, and Japanese Agricultural Stagnation: An Economic Consequence of Colonialism', *The Quarterly Journal of Economics*, LXXXIV/4 (1970), pp. 562–89.

27 Eckert, *Offsprings of Empire*, p. 41.

28 Cherl-ho Lee, 'Changes in the Dietary Patterns, Health, and Nutritional Status of Koreans During the Last Century', *Korean and Korean American Studies Bulletin*, VI/1 (1995), p. 34.

29 Chōsen sōtokufu shokusankyoku, ed., *Chōsen kōjō meibo: Shōwa 15 nenban* (Keijō, 1940).

30 Based on data ibid. and Chōsen sōtokufu shokusankyoku, ed., *Chōsen kōjō meibo: Shōwa 9 nenban* (Keijō, 1934).

31 Andrew J. Grajdanzev, *Modern Korea* (New York, 1944), p. 150.

32 Based on data in Chōsen sōtokufu, *Chōsen kōjō meibo: Shōwa 9 nenban* and Chōsen sōtokufu, *Chōsen kōjō meibo: Shōwa 15 nenban*.

33 Chōsen sōtokufu, *Chōsen kōjō meibo: Shōwa 9 nenban*, pp. 172, 178, 191.

34 Chōsen sōtokufu, *Chōsen kōjō meibo: Shōwa 15 nenban*, pp. 257, 261, 264, 265, 290, 308, 334, 338.

35 Katarzyna J. Cwiertka, 'From Yokohama to Amsterdam: Meidi-ya and Dietary Change in Modern Japan', in *Japanstudien 12: Essen und Ernährung im Modernen Japan*, ed. N. Liscutin and R. Haak (Munich, 2000), pp. 49–56.

36 Keijō shōkō kaigisho, ed., *Keijō kōjō ichiran* (Keijō, 1937), p. 58.

37 Han Pok-chin, *Uri Saenghwal paengnyŏn:ŭmsik* (Seoul, 2001), pp. 39–40.

38 Keijō, *Keijō kōjō ichiran*, pp. 57–61.

39 Nisshin seifun kabushiki kaisha shashi hensan iinkai, ed., *Nisshin seifun kabushiki kaisha shi* (Tokyo, 1955), pp. 188–91.

40 Morinaga seika kabushiki kaisha, *Morinaga gojûgo nenshi* (Tokyo, 1954), p. 328.

41 Meiji seika kabushiki kaisha, ed., *Meiji Seika no ayumi: Kau ki de tsukutte '60 nen, 1916–1976* (Tokyo, 1977), p. 18.

42 Joseph Alphonse Laker, 'Entrepreneurship and the Development of the Japanese Beer Industry, 1872–1937', PhD dissertation, Indiana University, Bloomington (1975), pp. 298–9; Kirin biiru kabushiki kaisha kōhōshitsu, ed., *Kirin biiru no rekishi, sengohen*, I (Tokyo, 1969), pp. 64–5.

43 Editorial, 'The Brewing Industry of Manchukuo', *Contemporary Manchuria*, 3 (1939), p. 73.

44 Kirin biiru kabushiki kaisha kōhōshitsu, ed., *Kirin biiru no rekishi, sengohen*, vol. I, p. 76; Laker, 'Entrepreneurship and the Development of the Japanese Beer Industry', pp. 293–4, 305–6.

45 Jack Goody, *Cooking, Cuisine and Class: A Study in Comparative Sociology* (Cambridge, 1982), p. 157.

46 Solomon H. Katz and William Woys Weaver, eds, *Encyclopedia of Food and Culture* (New York, 2003), vol. III, p. 29.

47 David Burton, *The Raj at Table* (London and Boston, 1993), pp. 68–71;

J.A.G. Roberts, *China to Chinatown: Chinese Food in the West* (London, 2002), pp. 66–70; Richard R. Wilk, 'Food and Nationalism: The Origins of "Belizean Food"', in *Food Nations: Selling Taste in Consumer Societies*, ed. W. Belasco and P. Scranton (New York and London, 2002), pp. 67–89.

48 Simon Naylor, 'Spacing the Can: Empire, Modernity, and the Globalisation of Food', *Environment and Planning*, A32 (2000), p. 1629.

49 Mark William Wilde, 'Industrialization of Food Processing in the United States, 1860–1960', PhD dissertation, University of Delaware, Newark (1988); Martin Bruegel, 'How the French Learned to Eat Canned Food, 1809–1930s', in *Food Nations*, ed. Belasco and Scranton, pp. 113–30.

50 Elsbeth Locher-Scholten, *Women and the Colonial State: Essays on Gender and Modernity in the Netherlands Indies, 1900–1942* (Amsterdam, 2000), pp. 141–6.

51 Cwiertka, *Modern Japanese Cuisine*, pp. 61–5.

52 Majima Ayu, 'Nikushoku to iu kindai: Meijiki Nihon ni okeru shokuniku gunji juyō to nikushokukan no tokuchō', *Ajia bunka kenkyū*, 11 (2002), p. 222.

53 Majima, 'Nikushoku to iu kindai', p. 225.

54 Cwiertka, *Modern Japanese Cuisine*, pp. 50–55, 152.

55 Niino Yutaka, 'An Introduction to Sources: The Agriculture and Forestry Bureau of the Government-General of Chōsen's General Plan of the Project to Increase Korean Beef, March 1938', paper presented at Chōsen kindai chiikishika kenkyûkai, Tokyo, 27 March 2006.

56 Shimokawa Harumi, 'Chōsen no kanzumegyō, I', *Shokugin chōsa geppō*, 62 (1943), pp. 19–22.

57 Ibid., pp. 22–4.

58 Hayashi Saburo, *Kōgun: The Japanese Army in the Pacific War* (Quantico, VA, 1959), pp. 8–20.

59 Shimokawa Harumi, 'Chōsen no kanzumegyō, II', *Shokugin chōsa geppō*, 63 (1943), p. 17.

60 Ibid., p. 3.

61 Shimokawa, 'Chōsen no kanzumegyō, I', pp. 8, 12.

62 Ibid., p. 10.

63 Yoshida Keiichi, *Chōsen suisan kaihatsu shi* (Shimonoseki, 1954), pp. 382, 388, 394.

64 Earl Chapin May, *The Canning Clan: A Pageant of Pioneering Americans* (New York, NY, 1937), p. 158.

65 Shimokawa, 'Chōsen no kanzumegyō, I', p. 9.

66 Ibid., pp. 13–14.

67 Shimokawa, 'Chōsen no kanzumegyō, II', pp. 3–4.

2 Consumption Colonized

1 Alain Delissen, 'Denied and Besieged: The Japanese of Korea, 1876–1945', in *New Frontiers: Imperialism's New Communities in East Asia, 1842–1953*, ed. R. Bickers and C. Henriot (Manchester, 2000), pp. 126–7.

2 Katarzyna J. Cwiertka, *Modern Japanese Cuisine: Food, Power and National Identity* (London, 2006), pp. 46–55.

3 Chŏn U-yong, 'Singminji tosi imiji wa munhwa hyŏnsang: 1920 nyŏndae ŭi Kyŏngsŏng?', in *Nikkan rekishi kyōdō kenkyū hōkokusho, dai san bunka hen jōkan*, ed. Nikkan rekishi kyōdō kenkyū iinkai (Tokyo, 2005), p. 9. Available at www.jkcf.or.jp (accessed 30 July 2010).

4 Kim Jin-song, *Sŏul e ttanssŭholŭl hŏhara: hyŏndaesŏngŭi hyŏngsŏng* (Seoul, 1999); Sin Myŏng-jik, *Modŏn boi Kyŏngsŏng ŭl kŏnilda* (Seoul, 2003); Yŏnse taehakkyo kukhak ycn'guwŏn, ed., *Ilche ŭi singmin chipae wa ilsang saenghwal* (Seoul, 2004).

5 Todd Andrew Henry, 'Keijō: Japanese and Korean Constructions of Colonial Seoul and the History of its Lived Spaces, 1910–1945', PhD dissertation, University of California, Los Angeles (2006), p. 56.

6 Henry, *Keijō*, p. 63.

7 Uchida Jun, '"Brokers of Empire": Japanese Settler Colonialism in Korea, 1910–1937', PhD dissertation, Harvard University, Cambridge, MA (2005); Nicole Cohen, 'Children of Empire: Growing up Japanese in Colonial Korea, 1876–1946', PhD dissertation, Columbia University, New York (2006).

8 Keijō shōkō kaigisho, *Keijō shōkō meiroku* (Keijō, 1939), pp. 252–69.

9 Keijō shōkō, *Keijō shōkō meiroku*, supplement, pp. 18–19.

10 Kwang-ok Kim, 'Contested Terrain of Imagination: Chinese Food in Korea', in *Changing Chinese Foodways in Asia*, ed. D.Y.H. Wu and C. B. Tan (Hong Kong, 2001), pp. 202–3; Young-kyun Yang, '*Jajangmyeon* and *Junggukjip:* The Changing Position and Meaning of Chinese Food and Chinese Restaurants in Korean Society', *Korea Journal*, XLV/2 (2005), p. 64.

11 Peter Duus, *The Abacus and the Sword: The Japanese Penetration of Korea, 1895–1910* (Berkeley, CA, 1995), pp. 324–8.

12 Chŏng Hye-kyŏng and Yi Chŏng-hye, *Sŏul e umsik munhwa: Yŏngyang hakkwa innyuhak e mannam* (Seoul, 1996), p. 96.

13 Yi Sŏng-u, 'Umsikchŏm', in *Han'guk minjok munhwa taebaekkwa sajŏn*, vol. XVII, ed. Han'guk chŏngsin munhwa yŏn'guwŏn p'yŏnch'anbu (Seoul, 1980), pp. 451–3; Kim Sang-bo, *Chosŏn sidaeŭi ŭmsik munhwa* (Seoul, 2006), pp. 152–73.

14 Andrei Lankov, *The Dawn of Modern Korea: The Transformation in Life and*

Cityscape (Seoul, 2007), pp. 164–5.

15 Yang, '*Jajangmyeon* and *Junggukjip*', p. 64.

16 Ibid., p. 65.

17 Ibid., p. 66.

18 Cwiertka, *Modern Japanese Cuisine*, pp. 42–55.

19 Ibid., p. 49.

20 Yi Yong-gi, *Chosŏn mubyŏn sinsik yori chebŏp* (Keijō, 1924), pp. 279–80.

21 Lankov, *The Dawn of Modern Korea*, p. 90.

22 Cwiertka, *Modern Japanese Cuisine*, pp. 39–41; Kim Won-mo, 'Misŭ Sont'ak kwa Sont'ak hot'el', *Hyangt'o Sŏul*, 56 (1996), p. 208.

23 Kim, 'Misŭ Sont'ak', pp. 208, 219.

24 Lankov, *The Dawn of Modern Korea*, p. 90.

25 Japan Tourist Bureau, *The Chōsen Hotel: Keijō (Seoul)* (n.p., n.d.), pp. 1–2.

26 T. Phillip Terry, *Terry's Guide to the Japanese Empire* (Boston and New York, 1933), p. 734.

27 Editorial, 'Shokudō haiken', *Chōsen oyobi Manshū*, 319 (1934), p. 87.

28 Ibid.

29 Terry, *Terry's Guide to the Japanese Empire*, p. 734; Yano Kanjō and Morikawa Seijin, *Shinhan dai Keijō annai* (Keijō, 1936), pp. 207–8.

30 Hyung-il Pai, 'Travel Guides to the Empire: The Production of Tourist Images in Colonial Korea', in *Consuming Korean Tradition in Early and Late Modernity*, ed. L. Kendall (Honolulu, HI, 2010), pp. 74–7.

31 Ariga Shin'ichirō, *Han'guk chiri p'ungsokchi ch'ongso, 42: Dai Keijō* (Seoul, 1990), p. 275.

32 Yano and Morikawa, *Shinhan dai Keijō annai*, pp. 207–8.

33 Ariga, *Dai Keijō*, pp. 363, 378.

34 Mun Il-p'yŏng, *Mun Il-p'yŏng 1934 nyŏn: Singminji sidae han chisigin ŭi ilgi* (P'aju, 2008).

35 Ibid.

36 Yŏm Sang-sŏp, *Three Generations* [1931, revd 1948], trans. Yu Young-nan (New York, 2005), pp. 45, 56, 77–8, 132–3, 136, 346.

37 Yi Sang, 'Wings' [1936], trans. Chu Yo-sup, in *Modern Korean Short Stories and Plays*, ed. Korean Centre International PEN (Seoul, 1970), pp. 211–12; Ch'ae Man-sik, 'A Ready-made Life' [1934], trans. Chong-un Kim and Bruce Dulton, in *A Ready-made Life: Early Masters of Modern Korean Fiction* (Honolulu, HI, 1998), p. 64.

38 Janet Poole, 'Colonial Interiors: Modernist Fiction of Korea', PhD dissertation, Columbia University, New York (2004), p. 41.

39 Yano and Morikawa, *Shinhan dai Keijō annai*, pp. 207–8.

40 Oh Jin-sŏk, 'Ilcheha paekkwajŏm ŏpke ŭi tonghyang kwa kwankeindŭl ŭi

saenghwal yangsik', in *Ilche ŭi singmin chipae wa ilsang saenghwal*, ed. Yŏnse taehakkyo kukhak yŏn'guwŏn (Seoul, 2004), p. 170; Kim T'ae-su, *Kkot kach'o p'iŏ maehokke hara* (Seoul, 2005), p. 253.

41 Editorial, 'Mitsukoshi, Chōjiya, Minakai shokudō gassenki', *Chōsen oyobi Manshū*, 317 (1934), p. 86.

42 Ibid., pp. 86–7.

43 Ibid., p. 87.

44 Erika D. Rappaport, '"A New Era of Shopping": The Promotion of Women's Pleasure in London's West End, 1909–1914', in *Cinema and the Invention of Modern Life*, ed. L. Charney and V. R. Schwartz (Berkeley, CA, 1995), p. 144.

45 William R. Leach, *Land of Desire: Merchants, Power, and the Rise of a New American Culture* (New York, 1993), p. 137.

46 See, for example, Kerrie L. MacPherson, ed., *Asian Department Stores* (Richmond, 1998), and Robert D. Tamilia, *The Wonderful World of the Department Store in Historical Perspective* (Montreal, 2002), at http://faculty.quinnipiac.edu (accessed 28 July 2010).

47 Rosalind H. Williams, *Dream Worlds: Mass Consumption in Late Nineteenth-century France* (Berkeley, CA, 1982), p. 91.

48 Kerrie L. MacPherson, 'Introduction: Asia's Universal Providers', in *Asian Department Stores*, ed. K. L. MacPherson (Richmond, Surrey, 1998), pp. 1–30.

49 Williams, *Dream Worlds*, p. 67.

50 Colin Campbell, 'The Desire for the New: Its Nature and Social Location as Presented in Theories of Fashion and Modern Consumerism', in *Consuming Technologies: Media and Information in Domestic Spaces*, ed. R. Silversone and E. Hirsch (London, 1992), pp. 48–62.

51 Leach, *Land of Desire*, p. 104.

52 Williams, *Dream Worlds*, p. 71.

53 MacPherson, 'Introduction', pp. 10–11.

54 Louise Young, 'Marketing the Modern: Department Stores, Consumer Culture, and the New Middle Class in Interwar Japan', *International Labor and Working Class History*, 55 (1999), p. 62.

55 Young, 'Marketing the Modern', p. 63.

56 Brian Moeran, 'The Birth of the Japanese Department Store', in *Asian Department Stores*, ed. MacPherson, p. 159.

57 Ibid., pp. 145–51.

58 Hayashi Hiroshige, *Maboroshi no Minakai hyakkaten: Chōsen o sekken shita Ômi shōnin hyakkaten no kōbō* (Tokyo, 2003), p. 99.

59 Matsuda Isao, *Watashi no rirekisho* (Tokyo, 1972), p. 26.

60 Hayashi, *Maboroshi no Minakai hyakkaten*, pp. 48–50.
61 Oh, 'Ilcheha paekkwajŏm ŏpke', pp. 130–33.
62 Hayashi, *Maboroshi no Minakai hyakkaten*, p. 175.
63 Oh, 'Ilcheha paekkwajŏm ŏpke', p. 137.
64 Hayashi, *Maboroshi no Minakai hyakkaten*, pp. 19, 105.
65 Inoue Shigeo, 'Keijō depāto gassen', *Chōsen oyobi Manshū*, 310 (1933), p. 81.
66 *Chosŏn Ilbo*, 11 November 1934, p. 4.
67 Oh, 'Ilcheha paekkwajŏm ŏpke', pp. 129–30; Poole, 'Colonial Interiors', p. 50.
68 Hayashi, *Maboroshi no Minakai hyakkaten*, pp. 149, 174–6.
69 *Samch'ŏlli*, October 1935, pp. 388–90, after Poole, 'Colonial Interiors', p. 50.
70 Williams, *Dream Worlds*, pp. 19–57.
71 Mica Nava, 'Modernity's Disavowal: Women, the City and the Department Store', in *Modern Times: Reflections on a Century of English Modernity*, ed. M. Nava and A. O'Shea (London, 1996), p. 46.
72 William R. Leach, 'Transformation in a Culture of Consumption: Women and Department Stores, 1890–1925', *The Journal of American History*, LXXI/2 (1984), p. 320.
73 *Chosŏn Ilbo*, 19 July 1930.
74 *Chosŏn Ilbo*, 19 July 1933.
75 Erika D. Rappaport, '"The Halls of Temptation": Gender, Politics, and the Construction of the Department Store in Late Victorian London', *The Journal of British Studies*, XXXV/1 (1996), p. 70.
76 Michael B. Miller, *The Bon Marché: Bourgeois Culture and the Department Store, 1869–1920* (London, 1981).
77 Rappaport, 'The Halls of Temptation', p. 71.
78 Ibid., p. 66.
79 Oh, 'Ilcheha paekkwajŏm ŏpke', pp. 142–3.
80 Yi, 'Umsikchŏm', pp. 451–3; *Chosŏn Chungang Ilbo*, 4 August 1934, after Poole, *Colonial Interiors*, p. 52.
81 Ralph M. Hower, *History of Macy's of New York, 1858–1919: Chapters in the Evolution of the Department Store* (Cambridge, MA, 1946), p. 161.
82 Leach, *Land of Desire*, p. 137.
83 See Sandra Mattielli, ed., *Virtues in Conflict: Tradition and the Korean Woman Today* (Seoul, 1977) for more information about the place of women in traditional Korean society and the changes brought about by modernization.
84 Kim, *Kkot kach'o p'iŏ maehokke hara*, pp. 257–8.
85 Mitsukoshi honsha, *Kabushiki kaisha Mitsukoshi 100 nen no kiroku* (Tokyo, 2005), p. 160.

86 *Chosŏn Ilbo*, 1 December 1934, p. 4.
87 Andrew J. Grajdanzev, *Modern Korea* (New York, 1944), pp. 180, 204.
88 Yi Kyŏng-hun, 'Missukkosi, kŭndae ŭi showindou: munhak kwa p'ungsok', in *Han'guk kŭndae munhak kwa Ilbon munhak*, ed. Han'guk munhak yŏn'gu hakhoe (Seoul, 2001), p. 118.

3 Industrializing Korean Taste

1 Although Korean has, phonologically, no distinction between voiced and voiceless consonants, it distinguishes them phonetically. Since the McCune-Reischauer romanization system followed in this book transcribes Korean words in the manner they are pronounced, the different pronunciation of the component '*chang*' in the word *kanjang*, *toenjang* and *koch'ujang* is reflected in their spelling.
2 Han Pong-nyŏ and Han Pok-chin, *Chongga chip siŏmŏni chang tamgŭnŭn pŏp* (Seoul, 1995), pp. 23–32; Yi Ch'un-ja et al., *Chang* (Seoul, 2003).
3 Katarzyna J. Cwiertka and Akiko Moriya, 'Fermented Soyfoods in South Korea: The Industrialization of Tradition', in *The World of Soy*, ed. C. Du Bois, C. B. Tan and S. Mintz (Urbana, IL, 2008), pp. 166–7. See also Han and Han, *Chongga chip siŏmŏni chang*, p. 24.
4 The National Academy of Korean Language, ed., *An Illustrated Guide to Korean Culture: 233 Traditional Key Words* (Seoul, 2002), pp. 65–8. See also Cornelius Osgood, *The Koreans and Their Culture* (New York, 1951), p. 86; and Cherl-ho Lee, *Fermentation Technology in Korea* (Seoul, 2001), p. 78.
5 Hi Soo Shin Hepinstall, *Growing Up in the Korean Kitchen: A Cookbook* (Berkeley, CA, 2001), p. xvi.
6 Nongsu ch'uksan sinmun, ed., *Hanguk sikp'um yŏn'gam* (Seoul, 2003), p. 348.
7 Peter Duus, *The Abacus and the Sword: The Japanese Penetration of Korea, 1895–1910* (Berkeley, CA, 1995), pp. 324–63.
8 Hirano Masaaki, 'Shōyu no rekishi: Sono yurai to hattatsu', in *Shōyu no hon*, ed. Tamura Heiji and Hirano Masaaki (Tokyo, 1971), pp. 30–45.
9 W. Mark Fruin, *Kikkoman: Company, Clan and Community* (Cambridge, MA, 1983), pp. 23–36.
10 Naomichi Ishige, *The History and Culture of Japanese Food* (London, 2001), pp. 114–15.
11 The manufacture of soy sauce according to the Korean method, the so-called *tamari shōyu*, continued in central Japan (Aichi, Mie and

Gifu prefectures). It was standard in Japan before the new method was introduced from China in the sixteenth century. See William Shurtleff and Akiko Aoyagi, 'History of Soy Sauce, Shoyu, and Tamari', in *History of Soybeans and Soyfoods: 1100 BC to the 1980s* (Lafayette, CA, 2007), at www.soyinfocenter.com (accessed 30 July 2010).

12 Hanai Shunsuke, 'Nōson chiiki chūshō shōyu jōzōka', in *Nihon no aji: Shōyu no rekishi*, ed. Hayashi Reiko and Amano Masatoshi (Tokyo, 2005), pp. 146–9.

13 Ioku Shigehiko, 'Fukuoka no shōyu no rekishi', in *Nihon no aji*, ed. Hayashi and Amano, p. 183. For a detailed analysis of geographical differences in home brewing see Nagatsuma Hiroshi, 'Kindai shōyu jōzōgyō to nōson', in *Shōyu jōzō gyōshi no kenkyū*, ed. Hayashi Reiko (Tokyo, 1990), pp. 430–32.

14 Tanaka Norio, *Shōyu kara sekai o miru* (Nagareyama, 1999), pp. 256–325.

15 Fruin, *Kikkoman*, pp. 72–5; Shurtleff and Aoyagi, 'History of Soy Sauce, Shoyu, and Tamari'.

16 Tanaka, *Shōyu kara sekai o miru*, p. 257.

17 Fruin, *Kikkoman*, p. 261.

18 Hanai, 'Nōson chiiki chūshō shōyu jōzōka', pp. 146–7.

19 Tanimoto Masayuki, 'Chōshi no shōyu jōzōgyō', in *Nihon no aji*, ed. Hayashi and Amano, pp. 107–9; Hanai, 'Nōson chiiki chūshō shōyu jōzōka', pp. 150–51, 158–9.

20 Liu Keshun, *Soybeans: Chemistry, Technology and Utilization* (Gaithersburg, MD, 1999), pp. 250–51.

21 Ajinomoto kabushiki kaisha, ed., *Ajinomoto enkakushi* (Tokyo, 1951), pp. 793–4.

22 Ōta Shizuyuki, *Umami chōmiryō no chishiki* (Tokyo, 1992), pp. 4–6.

23 P. H. Dorsett and William J. Morse, 'Agricultural Explorations in Japan, Chosen (Korea), Northeastern China, Taiwan (Formosa), Singapore, Java, Sumatra and Ceylon', unpublished manuscript, held in the National Archives, Washington, DC (1928–32), pp. 7066–7; Shikazono Naoharu and Yoshitaka Tomoda, 'Daizu kasu kasui bunkaibutsu (Soyamento) to shōyu no hikaku kenkyū', *Kōgyō Kagaku Zasshi*, 35 (1932), pp. 892–4; Dorothea Van Gundy, *La Sierra Recipes* (Ontario, 1936), p. 47.

24 Inoue Ayao, 'Shōyu', in *Shōwa no shokuhin sangyō shi*, ed. Nihon Shokuryō Shinbunsha (Tokyo, 1990), p. 489.

25 Marukin Shōyu of Shōdoshima in western Japan, for example, became a well-known brand of synthetic soy sauce. See Ajinomoto, *Ajinomoto enkakushi*, p. 794 and Fruin, *Kikkoman*, p. 261.

26 *Kyūsoku shokuryō taisaku ni kan suru ken. Kakugi kettei 26/09/1941*, available at www.ndl.go.jp (accessed 3 August 2010).

27 Ajinomoto, *Ajinomoto enkakushi*, appendix, p. 21.

28 Noda Shōyu acquired 80 per cent of Chōshi Shōyu shares in April 1937. The company grew three years later through the acquisition of Yamayama Shōyu. See Fruin, *Kikkoman*, p. 235; Ichiyama Morio, *Noda shōyu kabushiki kaisha nijūnen shi* (Noda, 1940), p. 679; and Noda shōyu kabushiki kaisha, ed., *Noda shōyu kabushiki kaisha sanjūnen shi* (Noda, 1955), p. 164.

29 Ajinomoto, *Ajinomoto enkakushi*, p. 797; Noda shōyu, *Noda shōyu*, p. 237.

30 Noda shōyu, *Noda shōyu*, pp. 236–7.

31 Inoue, 'Shōyu', p. 491; Noda shōyu, *Noda shōyu*, pp. 237–8.

32 Shurtleff and Aoyagi, 'History of Soy Sauce, Shoyu, and Tamari'.

33 Kikkoman (without the macron on the 'o') is the company's English name. The macron was retained when referring to Kikkōman as a brand of soy sauce.

34 Yokotsuka Tamotsu, *Nihon no shōyu: Sono genryū to kindai kōgyōka no kenkyū* (Tokyo, 2004), p. 101.

35 Ibid., pp. 25, 198.

36 Yi Han-ch'ang, *Chang: Yŏksa wa munhwa wa kong'ŏp* (Seoul, 1999), p. 159.

37 Ibid., p. 88; Taehan changnyu kong'ŏp hyŏptong chohap, ed., *Taehan changnyu kong'ŏp hyŏptong chohap 35 nyŏn sa* (Seoul, 1997), p. 56.

38 Yi, *Chang*, pp. 96–114.

39 Tsushima, 'Chōsen ni okeru miso oyobi shōyu jōzō no genjō ni tsuite', *Shokugin Chōsa Geppō*, 61 (1943), pp. 1–22; Tōkyō shiyakusho, ed., *Daitōa kyōeikennai ni okeru seikatsu hitsujuhin no jukyū to wariate sei* (Tokyo, 1943); Erich Pauer, 'Neighbourhood Associations and Food Distribution in Japanese Cities in World War II', in *Agriculture and Food Supply in the Second World War*, ed. B. Martin and A. S. Milward (Ostfildern, 1985), pp. 219–41.

40 Nagatsuma, 'Kindai shōyu jōzōgyō to nōson', p. 426.

41 In the early stages of settlement the vast majority of Japanese residents in Korea came from five prefectures, three in northern Kyushu (Nagasaki, Ōita, Fukuoka) and two in western Honshu (Yamaguchi and Hiroshima). See Duus, *The Abacus and the Sword*, p. 315.

42 Miyamoto Masayuki, *Chōsen shokuryōhin dōgyō hattatsushi* (Keijō, 1922), pp. 88–9.

43 Ichiyama, *Noda shōyu*, pp. 364–7; Duus, *The Abacus and the Sword*, p. 345.

44 Miyamoto, *Chōsen shokuryōhin*, p. 428; Yi, *Chang*, p. 110.

45 Yi, *Chang*, p. 98; Hayashi Reiko, 'Kaigai de no seisan to shōhi', in *Nihon no aji*, ed. Hayashi and Amano, pp. 44–5.

46 Ichiyama, *Noda shōyu*, p. 364.

47 Keijō shōkō kaigisho, ed., *Keijō ni okeru kōjō chōsa* (Keijō, 1937), p. 89.

48 Tsushima, 'Chōsen ni okeru miso oyobi shōyu', p. 12. The figure is much higher than the 22, 72 and 69 respectively calculated by other sources only a few years earlier. See Nakamura Sukeyoshi, ed., *Chōsen ginkō kaisha kumiai yōroku fukyūhan* (Keijō, 1940); Chōsen sōtokufu shokusankyoku, ed., *Chōsen kōjō meibo: Shōwa 15 nenban* (Keijō, 1940); and Taehan changnyu, *Taehan changnyu kong'ŏp*, p. 63. A possible explanation is that Tsushima, under wartime mobilization and controlled distribution of resources, was able to count all manufacturers, while company registers published earlier did not include very small businesses. Even considering this margin, war's stimulation of the soy sauce industry in colonial Korea remains unquestionable.

49 Tsushima, 'Chōsen ni okeru miso oyobi shōyu', p. 13.

50 Nagatsuma, 'Kindai shōyu jōzōgyō to nōson', pp. 444–6.

51 Hayashi Reiko, 'Shōyu no genryō', in *Nihon no aji*, ed. Hayashi Reiko and Amano Masatoshi (Tokyo, 2005), p. 33; Tsushima, 'Chōsen ni okeru miso oyobi shōyu', p. 3.

52 Tsushima, 'Chōsen ni okeru miso oyobi shōyu', p. 10.

53 Jung-en Woo, *Race to the Swift: State and Finance in Korean Industrialization* (New York, 1991), pp. 35–6.

54 Yun Myŏng-hŏng, '"Sangyō concern" to shite no Chōsen Chisso', in *Chōsen ni okeru Nitchitsu concern*, ed. Kang Chae-ŏn (Tokyo, 1985), p. 244.

55 Barbara Molony, *Technology and Investment: The Prewar Japanese Chemical Industry* (Cambridge, MA, 1990), p. 234.

56 Ajinomoto, *Ajinomoto enkakushi*, p. 441.

57 Chōsen sōtokufu shokusankyoku, ed., *Chōsen kōjō meibo: Shōwa 18 nenban* (Keijō, 1943), pp. 413–14.

58 David Wolff, 'Bean There: Toward a Soy-based History of Northeast Asia', *The South Atlantic Quarterly*, XCIX/1 (2000), pp. 241–52; Molony, *Technology and Investment*, p. 234.

59 Ichiyama, *Noda shōyu*, pp. 674–6.

60 Noda shōyu, *Noda shōyu*, p. 233.

61 Hayashi, 'Kaigai de no seisan to shōhi', pp. 40–43.

62 Hochin Choi, 'The Strengthening of the Economic Domination by Japanese Colonialism (1932–1945): Statistical Analysis', *Yŏnsei Nonch'ong*, 7 (1969), p. 361.

63 Yi mentions only one Korean-owned brewery, capitalized with 25,000 yen and employing three workers. It is possible that this enterprise was Heijō Shōyu Co., established in Pyongyang in 1926. See Yi, *Chang*, pp. 98–9; Teikoku kyōshinjo, *Teikoku ginkō kaisha yōroku* (Tokyo, 1927), p. 7; and Nakamura Sukeyoshi, ed., *Chōsen ginkō kaisha kumiai yōroku fukyūhan* (Keijō, 1931), p. 176.

64 Chōsen, *Chōsen kōjō meibo: Shōwa 15 nenban*, p. 254; Chōsen, *Chōsen kōjō meibo: Shōwa 18 nenban*, p. 414. See also www.monggofood.co.kr (accessed 3 August 2010).

65 Yi, *Chang*, p. 97.

66 Keijō shōkō kaigisho, *Keijō ni okeru kōjō chōsa*, p. 80.

67 Miyamoto, *Chōsen shokuryōhin*, p. 428; Hayashi, 'Kaigai de no seisan to shōhi', p. 45.

68 Fruin, *Kikkoman*, p. 236; Hayashi, 'Kaigai de no seisan to shōhi', p. 42.

69 Tsushima, 'Chōsen ni okeru miso oyobi shōyu', p. 18.

70 See Dennis L. McNamara, *Trade and Transformation in Korea, 1876–1945* (Boulder, CO, 1998); Soon-won Park, *Colonial Industrialization and Labor in Korea* (Cambridge, MA, 1999); and Morita Yoshio and Kanako Osada, *Kita chōsen chiiki Nihonjin no hikiage* (Tokyo, 1980).

71 Allan K. Smith, *Oriental Methods of Using Soybeans as Food with Special Attention to Fermented Products* (Washington, DC, 1949), p. 37.

72 Jong-Won Lee, 'The Impact of the Korean War on the Korean Economy', *International Journal of Korean Studies*, V/1 (2001), pp. 97–118.

73 See 'History', at www.monggofood.co.kr.

74 Chōsen, *Chōsen kōjō meibo: Shōwa 18 nenban*, p. 410.

75 Seamp'yo Sikp'um, *Saemp'yo sikp'um ŭi yŏksa: Chaepum, sŏlbi chungsim.* Internal publication of Seamp'yo Sikp'um (Seoul, year of publication unknown), pp. 1–2. Interestingly, the colonial origins are not disclosed on the company's public website. See www.sempio.com (accessed 3 August 2010).

76 See www.meilfood.com (accessed 16 April 2012).

77 Taehan changnyu, *Taehan changnyu kong'ŏp*, pp. 81–3.

78 Nongsu ch'uksan sinmun, *Hanguk sikp'um yŏn'gam*, p. 343.

79 Yi, *Chang*, p. 159. For specific information on different types of industrial soy sauce and their names see Yi Ch'un-ja et al., *Chang*, p. 49.

80 The Korean Nutrition Society, *Korean Nutrition Resources Data* (Seoul, 1989), pp. 223–4.

81 Doo-sub Kim and Cheong-seok Kim, *The Population of Korea* (Taejeon, 2004), p. 333.

82 Woo, *Race to the Swift*, p. 41.

83 Sidney W. Mintz, *Sweetness and Power: The Place of Sugar in Modern History* (New York, 1985).
84 Kim Ŭng-dŏk et al., ed., *Han'guk kwanggo 100 nyŏn, ha* (Seoul, 1996), p. 11.
85 Saemp'yo Sikp'um, *'Kanjang' hamyŏn paro kŭ irŭm Saemp'yo: Saemp'yo kanjang ŭi yŏksa*. Internal publication of Saemp'yo Sikp'um (Seoul, year of publication unknown), pp. 4–5.
86 Jordan Sand, 'A Short History of MSG: Good Science, Bad Science, and Taste Cultures', *Gastronomica*, V/4 (2005), p. 38.
87 Ibid., p. 42.
88 Ibid., p. 42. See also Karl Gerth, *China Made: Consumer Culture and the Creation of the Nation* (Cambridge, MA, 2003), pp. 341–5.
89 Ajinomoto, *Ajinomoto enkakushi*, pp. 436–40.
90 Ibid., p. 512.
91 Ibid., p. 441.
92 Keun-sik Jung, 'Colonial Modernity and the Social History of Chemical Seasoning in Korea', *Korea Journal*, XLV/2 (2005), pp. 22–3.
93 Jung, 'Colonial Modernity and the Social History of Chemical Seasoning in Korea', p. 26.
94 Ibid., p. 29.
95 Ibid., pp. 33–4.
96 Yokotsuka, *Nihon no shōyu*, p. 159.

4 Wartime Food Management and Its Legacy

1 Helie Lee, *Still Life with Rice: A Young American Woman Discovers the Life and Legacy of Her Korean Grandmother* (New York, 1996), p. 230.
2 Fujiwara Akira, *Uejini shita eireitachi* (Tokyo, 2001), p. 3.
3 Nguyên Thê Anh, 'Japanese Food Policies and the 1945 Great Famine in Indochina', in *Food Supplies and the Japanese Occupation in South-east Asia*, ed. P. Kratoska (New York, 1998), pp. 214–18.
4 George M. McCune, *Korea Today* (Cambridge, MA, 1950), pp. 121–2.
5 This observation is based on a pilot study conducted by the author in Seoul in the winter of 2005.
6 Jong-Won Lee, 'The Impact of the Korean War on the Korean Economy', *International Journal of Korean Studies*, V/1 (2001), pp. 97–118.
7 Allan R. Millet, *The War for Korea, 1945–1950: A House Burning* (Lawrence, KS, 2005), pp. 52–3.
8 A meticulous description of the developments leading to the Korean

War can be found in Bruce Cumings, *The Origins of the Korean War*, vol. I: *Liberation and the Emergence of Separate Regimes, 1945–1947* (Princeton, NJ, 1981) and vol. II: *The Roaring of the Cataract, 1947–1950* (Princeton, NJ, 1990). For a more concise version of the story see Millet, *The War for Korea* and Stanley Sandler, *The Korean War: No Victors, No Vanquished* (London, 1999).

9 A full text of the armistice agreement can be found at http://news.findlaw.com (accessed 10 August 2010).

10 Bruce Cumings, *The Korean War: A History* (New York, 2010), pp. 35, 159–60, 243.

11 Ina Zweiniger-Bargielowska and Rachel Duffett, eds, *Food and War in Twentieth-Century Europe* (Farnham, 2011). See also Katarzyna J. Cwiertka, ed., *Food and War in Mid-Twentieth-Century East Asia* (Farnham, forthcoming).

12 See George Ginsburgs, *Soviet Works on Korea, 1945–1970* (Los Angeles, CA, 1973); Lester H. Brune, ed., *The Korean War: Handbook of the Literature and Research* (Westport, CT, 1996).

13 See Eui-hang Shin, 'Effects of the Korean War on Social Structures of the Republic of Korea: A Socio-demographic Analysis', *California Sociologist*, 15 (1992), pp. 21–42; Han'guk chŏngsin munhwa yŏn'guwŏn, ed., *Han'guk chŏnjaeng kwa sahoe kujo ŭi pyŏnhwa* (Seoul, 1999); Special issue of *Asia munhwa*, 16 (2000) on the Korean War and cultural change; Kyŏngsang taehakkyo sahoe kwahak yŏn'guso, ed., *Han'guk chŏnjaeng gwa Han'guk chabonjuŭi* (Seoul, 2000); Special issue of the *International Journal of Korean Studies*, V/1 (2001); Yi Dae-gŭn, *Haebanghu–1950 nyŏndae ŭi kyŏngje: Kong'ŏphwa ŭi sajŏk paegyŏng yŏn'gu* (Seoul, 2002).

14 See Donald K. Chung, *The Three Day Promise: A Korean Soldier's Memoir* (Tallahassee, FL, 1989); Ahn Junghyo, *Silver Stallion: A Novel of Korea* (New York, 1990); Pak Wan-so, trans. Yu Young-nan, *The Naked Tree* (Ithaca, NY, 1995); Lee, *Still Life with Rice*; Philip West and Chi-mun So, eds, *Remembering the 'Forgotten War': The Korean War Through Literature and Art* (Armonk, NY, 2001); Patrick Dowdey, ed., *Living Through the Forgotten War: Portrait of Korea* (Middletown, CT, 2004).

15 Chung, *The Three Day Promise*, p. 48.

16 Lee, *Still Life with Rice*, pp. 248–9.

17 The author's name has been romanized in many different ways, of which Park Wan-suh and Pak Wan-so are the most common.

18 Park Wan-suh, trans. Yu Young-nan and Stephen J. Epstein, *Who Ate Up All the Shinga? An Autobiographical Novel* (New York, 2009),

pp. 139, 142.

19 Ibid., p. 141.

20 Ibid., p. 231.

21 Ibid., p. 248.

22 Hwang Sunwŏn, trans. Bruce and Ju-chan Fulton, 'The Toad', in *Lost Souls: Stories* (New York, 2010), p. 163.

23 Ibid., pp. 160–61, 184.

24 Carol Gluck, 'The Past in the Present', in *Postwar Japan as History*, ed. Andrew Gordon (Berkeley, CA, 1992), p. 76.

25 Bruce F. Johnston with Mosaburo Hosoda and Yoshio Kusumi, *Japanese Food Management in World War II* (Stanford, CA, 1953); Jerome B. Cohen, *Japan's Economy in War and Reconstruction* (Minneapolis, MN, 1949), pp. 364–86.

26 Erich Pauer, 'Introduction', in *Japan's War Economy*, ed. E. Pauer (London, 1999), pp. 1–8; Katarzyna J. Cwiertka, 'Militarization of Nutrition in Wartime Japan', *IIAS Newsletter*, 38 (2005), p. 15; Katarzyna J. Cwiertka, 'Western Food and the Making of the Japanese Nation-state', in *The Politics of Food*, ed. M. E. Lien and B. Nerlich (Oxford and New York, 2004), pp. 130–35.

27 Chōsen sōtokufu, *Chōsen sōtokufu shisei nenpō* (Keijō, 1942), pp. 270–71.

28 Johnston, *Japanese Food Management*, p. 181.

29 Ibid., pp. 191–8; Cohen, *Japan's Economy in War and Reconstruction*, p. 373; Howard F. Smith, 'Food Controls in Occupied Japan', *Agricultural History*, XXIII/3 (1949), p. 221.

30 For details concerning the Japanese food rationing system see Cohen, *Japan's Economy in War and Reconstruction*, pp. 374–9; Johnston, *Japanese Food Management*, pp. 165–212; and Erich Pauer, 'A New Order for Japanese Society: Planned Economy, Neighbourhood Associations and Food Distribution in Japanese Cities in the Second World War', in *Japan's War Economy*, ed. E. Pauer (London, 1999), pp. 89–102.

31 Johnston, *Japanese Food Management*, pp. 150, 204. *Gō* refers to a traditional Japanese unit of volume, nearly equal to the Korean *hop* (1 *hop* = 0.99 *gō*), equivalent to 0.18 litre.

32 'Shokuryō kanri hō Chōsen shikō rei no kōfu', *Jinkō mondai kenkyū*, III/7 (1942), p. 33, available at www.ipss.go.jp (accessed 11 August 2010).

33 Johnston, *Japanese Food Management*, p. 137.

34 'Chōsen shokuryō kanri rei no kōfu', *Jinkō mondai kenkyū*, IV/9 (1943), p. 55, available at www.ipss.go.jp (accessed 11 August 2010).

35 John W. Masland, 'Neighborhood Associations in Japan', *Far Eastern Survey*, XV/23 (1946), p. 355; Ralph J. D. Braibanti, 'Neighborhood

Associations in Japan and Their Democratic Potentialities', *The Far Eastern Quarterly*, VII/2 (1948), p. 151; Pauer, 'A New Order for Japanese Society', p. 95.

36 *Handbook for Village and Neighborhood Ration Boards: Special Explanation of Rice Ration Books in Tokyo-fu*. US Strategic Bombing Survey; Microfilm M1652, roll 61; RG 243, National Archives at College Park, College Park, Maryland.

37 Michael E. Robinson, *Korea's Twentieth-Century Odyssey: A Short History* (Honolulu, HI, 2007), p. 96; Kyoung-hee Park, '"Patriotic Unit" (*aegukpan*) as Wartime Legacy: Food Rationing in Korea During the Asia-Pacific War (1937–1945)'. Paper presented at the Graduate Student Convention in Korean Studies, Cluj-Napoca, 28 July 2010. See also chapter 2 in Kyoung-hee Park, 'State and Food in South Korea: Moulding National Diet in Wartime and Beyond (1937–1976)', PhD dissertation, Leiden University (forthcoming).

38 *Chosŏn Ilbo*, 25 April 1940, p. 2; Yi Chong-min, 'Chŏnsi ha aegukpan chochik kwa tosi ŭi ilsang t'ongje: Kyŏngsŏngbu rŭl chungsim ŭro', *Tongbang Hakchi*, 124 (2004), pp. 846–7, after Park, 'Patriotic Unit'.

39 Yi, 'Chŏnsi ha aegukpan chochik kwa tosi ŭi ilsang t'ongje', p. 873.

40 *Bunkyō no Chōsen*, 176 (1940), pp. 23–4.

41 Park, 'State and Food in South Korea', chapter 2.

42 Hŏ Yŏng-nan, 'Chŏnsi ch'echegi (1937–1945) saenghwal p'ilsup'um paegŭp t'ongje yŏn'gu', *Kuksakwan Nonch'ong*, 88 (2000), p. 321.

43 Kim Yŏng-mi, 'Ilche sigi Han'guk chŏnchaenggi chumin tongwŏn, t'ongje yŏn'gu: Sŏul chiyŏk chŏng, donghoe chochik pyŏnhwa rŭl chungsim ŭro', PhD dissertation, Seoul National University (2005), p. 72, after Park, 'Patriotic Unit'.

44 Kim In-ho, 'Taep'yŏngyang chŏnjaeng sigi: Sŏul chiyŏk ŭi sengp'ilp'um paegŭp t'ongje silt'ae', *Sŏulhak Yŏn'gu*, XXVI (2006), p. 103.

45 Keijō shōkō kaigisho, ed., *Chōsen ni okeru busshi no haikyū tōsei to haikyū kikō* (Keijō, 1943).

46 Ibid., p. 41.

47 McCune, *Korea Today*, p. 103.

48 Robinson, *Korea's Twentieth-Century Odyssey*, p. 105.

49 USAMGIK National Economic Board, *Food Position Report for South Korea*, December 1946–30 November 1948 (Seoul, 1947), p. 2. Box 8395, RG 331, National Archives at College Park, College Park, Maryland.

50 Pu Mi-sŏn, '1945–46 nyŏn migunjŏng ŭi migok sijang chayu chŏngch'aek', MA dissertation, Sŏgang University, Seoul (2002).

51 Cumings, *The Origins of the Korean War*, vol. I, p. 202.

52 Robinson, *Korea's Twentieth-Century Odyssey*, pp. 105–7; Cumings, *The Korean War*, pp. 109–11.

53 McCune, *Korea Today*, p. 104.

54 Cumings, *The Origins of the Korean War*, vol. 1, p. 375.

55 Ibid., p. 204.

56 USAMGIK, *Food Position Report for South Korea*, p. 4.

57 Cumings, *The Origins of the Korean War*, vol. 1, p. 378.

58 *Republic of Korea Statistics Summation*, 15 (March 1950), p. 95.

59 South Korean Interim Government, National Economic Board, *Annual Report USAMGIK Service of Civilian Supply for 1947* (Seoul, 1948). Box 98, RG 331, National Archives at College Park, College Park, Maryland.

60 A traditional Korean unit of volume, 1 *hop* is nearly equal to the Japanese *gō* (1 *hop* = 0.99 *gō*), 0.18 litre.

61 USAMGIK National Food Administration, *The Food Position of South Korea as of 1 May 1946*, p. 1. Box 8398, RG 331, National Archives at College Park, College Park, Maryland. See also Cumings, *The Origins of the Korean War*, vol. 1, p. 204.

62 South Korean Interim Government, National Economic Board, *Food and Agriculture Situation in Korea, 1948–1949* (Seoul, 1948), p. 45. Box 8843, RG 331, National Archives at College Park, College Park, Maryland.

63 National Economic Board, *Food and Agriculture Situation in Korea*, pp. 46–8.

64 USAMGIK, *The Food Position of South Korea as of 1 May 1946*, p. 1.

65 *Republic of Korea Statistics Summation*, 13 (January 1950), p. 16.

66 National Economic Board, *Food and Agriculture Situation in Korea*, pp. 11, 20.

67 Kim Hak-jae, '1950 nyŏndae kukkagwŏnnyŏk kwa haengchŏng maldan kigu: Kungminban ŭl t'ong han kamsi wa ton'wŏn', *Yŏksa Yŏn'gu*, 24 (2004), pp. 155–61.

68 Ibid., pp. 161–79, 183, 189.

69 Kyoung-hee Park, 'Daily Life Improvement Campaigns and the Korean War', in *Association for Korean Studies in Europe Proceedings of the 24th Biennial Conference*, ed. K. de Ceuster and M.C. van den Haak (Leiden, 2009).

70 Kim, '1950 nyŏndae kukkagwŏnnyŏk kwa haengchŏng maldan kigu', p. 174–5. See also Park, 'Daily Life Improvement Campaigns'.

71 McCune, *Korea Today*, p. 343.

72 USAMGIK, *Food Position Report for South Korea*, pp. 3–4.

73 USAMGIK, Disposal of Deteriorated Subsistence, letter of J. W. Fraser to Commanding General USAMGIK, 2 December 1947. Box 92,

RG 554, National Archives at College Park, College Park, Maryland.

74 Ahn, *Silver Stallion*, pp. 49, 79–80, 83, 109, 131; Pak Wan-so, *The Naked Tree*, p. 13.

75 Sahr Conway-Lanz, 'Beyond No Gun Ri: Refugees and the United States Military in the Korean War', *Diplomatic History*, XXIX/1 (2005), p. 50. See also Janice Kim, 'Between Mountains: Refugee Life During the Korean War, 1948–1960', in *Association for Korean Studies in Europe Proceedings of the 24th Biennial Conference*, ed. K. de Ceuster and M. C. van den Haak (Leiden, 2009).

76 Sahr Conway-Lanz, 'Beyond No Gun Ri', pp. 74–5.

77 Charles K. Armstrong, *The North Korean Revolution, 1945–1950* (Ithaca, NY, 2003), pp. 46–7.

78 Ibid., pp. 143–4.

79 Catherine Merridale, *Ivan's War: The Red Army, 1939–1945* (London, 2005), pp. 277–8. Looting practices on the Western front are described in detail on pp. 93, 103–4, 115–16, 277–82.

80 Park, *Who Ate Up All the Shinga?*, p. 164.

81 Armstrong, *The North Korean Revolution*, p. 143.

82 A *chŏngbo* is a Korean unit of land measurement (one *chŏngbo* translates to approximately 2.45 acres or 0.99 hectares); Mun Woong Lee, 'Rural North Korea Under Communism: A Study of Socio-cultural Change', PhD dissertation, Rice University, Houston, Texas (1975), p. 19.

83 Lee, 'Rural North Korea', pp. 22–3.

84 Armstrong, *The North Korean Revolution*, pp. 146–7.

85 Ibid., p. 146 note 44 and p. 165 note 145.

86 Ibid., pp. 77, 144.

87 Lee, 'Rural North Korea', pp. 20–21, 24.

88 McCune, *Korea Today*, p. 132. See also C. Clyde Mitchell, 'Land Reform in South Korea', *Pacific Affairs*, XXII/2 (1949), pp. 144–54.

89 Cumings, *The Origins of the Korean War*, vol. II, p. 472.

90 Armstrong, *The North Korean Revolution*, pp. 148–9.

91 United States Department of State, *North Korea: A Study in the Techniques of Takeover* (Washington, DC, 1961), p. 57, after Armstrong, *The North Korean Revolution*, p. 75.

92 Suk Lee, 'Food Shortages and Economic Institutions in the Democratic People's Republic of Korea', PhD dissertation, University of Warwick (2003), p. 49, available at http://wrap.warwick.ac.uk (accessed 2 September 2011).

93 Ibid., p. 60.

94 Armstrong, *The North Korean Revolution*, p. 144.

95 Lee, 'Food Shortages and Economic Institutions', p. 62.

96 Charles R. Shrader, *Communist Logistics in the Korean War* (Westport, CT, 1995), pp. 69, 94.

97 Ibid., p. 63.

98 Ibid., p. 94.

99 Mark R. Jacobson, '"Minds Then Hearts": U.S. Political and Psychological Warfare During the Korean War', PhD dissertation, Ohio State University, Columbus (2005), pp. 100–03.

100 Far East Command, Psychological Warfare Section, First Radio Broadcasting and Leaflet Group, Leaflet Food Thomo 1122 (Comp. Lflt 7102), 23 October 1951.

101 Far East Command, Psychological Warfare Section, First Radio Broadcasting and Leaflet Group, Leaflet Don't Starve This Winter 1230*, 28 October 1952; Far East Command, Psychological Warfare Section, First Radio Broadcasting and Leaflet Group, Leaflet Hide Your Rice 1232, 25 October 1952.

102 Jacobson, '"Minds Then Hearts"', pp. 96–7.

103 Jake Lyons, 'Feeding the United Nations in Korea', *The Quartermaster Review*, XXXI/1 (1951), p. 7.

104 R. G. Norman, 'Unique Operations Tokyo Quartermaster Depot', *The Quartermaster Review*, XXXI/4 (1952), p. 24.

105 Coy W. Baldwin, 'Food Service United Nations', *The Quartermaster Review*, XXXII/6 (1953), p. 117.

106 Chung, *The Three Day Promise*, p. 222.

107 James A. Huston, *Guns and Butter, Powder and Rice: U.S. Army Logistics in the Korean War* (London and Toronto, 1989), p. 123.

108 Lyons, 'Feeding the United Nations in Korea', pp. 7, 151.

109 Gregg Brazinsky, *Nation Building in South Korea: Koreans, Americans, and the Making of Democracy* (Chapel Hill, NC, 2007), pp. 72–8.

110 Cumings, *The Korean War*, p. 42; Ernest J. Skroch, 'Quartermaster Advisors in Korea', *The Quartermaster Review*, XXXI/2 (1951), pp. 8–9, 123.

111 Fujita Masao, *Shashin de miru Nihon rikugun heiei no shokuji* (Tokyo, 2009), pp. 27–9, 48–9.

112 Leonard G. Zewen, 'QM Developments in ROK Army', *The Quartermaster Review*, XXXIII/6 (1954), pp. 22–3, 120.

113 Huston, *Guns and Butter*, p. 339.

114 Chung, *The Three Day Promise*, p. 217. For more accounts of food shortages in the ROK army see pp. 181, 189.

115 Alex N. Williams, 'Subsistence Supply in Korea', *The Quartermaster Review*, XXXII/4 (1953), p. 29.

116 Ibid., p. 30.
117 Editorial, 'News from Overseas: Fresh Food for the Troops', *The Quartermaster Review*, XXXII/1 (1952), p. 21.
118 Williams, 'Subsistence Supply in Korea', p. 29.
119 Cecil W. Hospelhorn, 'Airborne Quartermasters', *The Quartermaster Review*, XXXIV/2 (1954), p. 16; Huston, *Guns and Butter*, p. 194.
120 Huston, *Guns and Butter*, pp. 339–40.
121 Ibid., p. 195.
122 Extract from Skroch, 'Quartermaster Advisors in Korea', p. 121.
123 Kawashima Shirō, 'Kankokugun no taberu keitai kōryō', *Bungei Shunjū*, XXIX/13 (1951), pp. 16–19.
124 Norman, 'Unique Operations Tokyo Quartermaster Depot', pp. 24, 112–13.

5 South Korea: From Food Aid to the Revival of Royal Cuisine

1 Ahn Junghyo, *Silver Stallion: A Novel of Korea* (New York, 1990), p. 141.
2 The Korea Foundation, ed., *The Korean Food Guide in English* (Seoul, 2003), p. 76.
3 James A. Huston, *Guns and Butter, Powder and Rice: U.S. Army Logistics in the Korean War* (London and Toronto, 1989), p. 123.
4 Ji-yeon Yuh, *Beyond the Shadow of Camptown: Korean Military Brides in America* (New York, 2002), pp. 20–21. See also Katharine H. S. Moon, *Sex among Allies: Military Prostitution in U.S.–Korea Relations* (New York, 1997).
5 Yuh, *Beyond the Shadow of Camptown*, p. 22.
6 Pak Wan-so, trans. Yu Young-nan, *The Naked Tree* (Ithaca, NY, 1995).
7 *The Korean Republic*, 9 September 1953.
8 The Korean Reconstruction Bank, ed., *Industry in Korea: 1967* (Seoul, 1967), pp. 101–3.
9 Laura Nelson, *Measured Excess: Status, Gender, and Consumer Nationalism in South Korea* (New York, 2000), pp. 6, 10.
10 Gregg Brazinsky, *Nation Building in South Korea: Koreans, Americans, and the Making of Democracy* (Chapel Hill, NC, 2007), p. 38.
11 Seungsook Moon, *Militarized Modernity and Gendered Citizenship in South Korea* (Durham, NC, 2005), p. 2.
12 Moon, *Militarized Modernity*, pp. 9–11.
13 Nelson, *Measured Excess*, pp. 6, 14.
14 Paul W. Kuznets, 'Causes, Consequences, Relevance: Korea's Industrialization', in *Transformations in Twentieth-Century Korea*,

ed. Chang Yun-shik and Steven Hugh Lee (London, 2006), pp. 92–7. See also Nelson, *Measured Excess*, pp. 10–18.

15 Remco Breuker, 'Korea's Forgotten War: Appropriating and Subverting the Vietnam War in Korean Popular Imaginings', *Korean Histories*, I/1 (2009), p. 40, available online at koreanhistories.net. See also Richard Stubbs, *Rethinking Asia's Economic Miracle: The Political Economy of War, Prosperity and Crisis* (New York, 2005), pp. 133–6.

16 Moon, *Militarized Modernity*, pp. 17–43, 78–80.

17 Larry L. Burmeister, 'Agricultural Cooperative Development and Change: A Window on South Korea's Agrarian Transformation', in *Transformations in Twentieth-Century Korea*, ed. Chang and Lee (London, 2006), p. 70.

18 *Chosŏn Ilbo*, 25 January 1969, after Kyoung-hee Park, 'Kankoku oyobi Nihon ni okeru shokuseikatsu no henka to sono tokuchō: Kakushu tōkei shiryō no bunseki o chūshin ni', MA dissertation, Tokyo Kasei-Gakuin University (2005), pp. 32–3. See also Moon, *Militarized Modernity*, p. 68.

19 Korean Reconstruction Bank, ed., *Industry in Korea*, pp. 98–9; Chae Kung Oh, *The Handbook of Korea* (New York, 1958), p. 219.

20 Editorial, 'Pingon kwa p'ungyo ŭi okkallim punsik kwa pulgogi', *Hyangt'o wa munhwa*, XXIII (August 2002), p. 74.

21 The Korean Nutrition Society, *Korean Nutrition Resource Data* (Seoul, 1989), p. 248.

22 Ibid., p. 28; Park, 'Kankoku oyobi Nihon ni okeru', pp. 26–7. See also Nelson, *Measured Excess*, pp. 74–5; Han'guk oesik chŏngbo, *Han'guk oesik yŏn'gam* (Seoul, 2009), p. 387.

23 Park, 'Kankoku oyobi Nihon ni okeru', pp. 33–4.

24 Nongsim kŭrup, *Nongsim 40 nyŏnsa* (Seoul, 2006), p. 305.

25 Han'guk sikp'um kong'ŏp hyŏphoe, *Sikp'um kong'ŏp hyŏphoe 30 nyŏnsa, 1969–1999* (Seoul, 2000), pp. 107–8.

26 '10 Consumer Hits 1950–2007', *Korea Times*, 16 October 2007, at www.koreatimes.co.kr (accessed 20 August 2010).

27 'Instant Ramen', at www.instantramen.or.jp (accessed 2 September 2011).

28 Han Kyŏng-ŏn, 'Hanguk ŭi sahoe pyŏndong e ttarŭn sikp'um sugŭp mit siksaenghwal haengdong pyŏnhwa e kwan han yŏn'gu: 1960 nyŏndae ihu ŭi munhŏn yŏn'gu rŭl chungsim ŭro', MA dissertation, Chungang University, Seoul (1990). After Park, 'Kankoku oyobi Nihon ni okeru', p. 48.

29 Katarzyna J. Cwiertka, *Modern Japanese Cuisine: Food, Modernity and National Identity* (London, 2006), pp. 144–7. See also George Solt, 'Ramen and U.S. Occupation Policy', in *Japanese Foodways, Past and*

Present, ed. Eric C. Rath and Stephanie Assmann (Champaign, IL, 2010), pp. 186–200.

30 Korean Reconstruction Bank, ed., *Industry in Korea,* pp. 85–6.

31 Korean Nutrition Society, *Korean Nutrition Resource Data*, p. 164.

32 Park, 'Kankoku oyobi Nihon ni okeru', pp. 42–3.

33 Han Kyung-koo, 'Noodle Odyssey: East Asia and Beyond', *Korea Journal*, L/1 (2010), p. 68.

34 Park, 'Kankoku oyobi Nihon ni okeru', pp. 25–9.

35 Korean Nutrition Society, *Korean Nutrition Resource Data*, p. 27.

36 Vincent S. R. Brandt, *A Korean Village: Between Farm and Sea* (Cambridge, MA, 1971), p. 51.

37 Clark W. Sorensen, *Over the Mountains Are Mountains: Korean Peasant Households and Their Adaptations to Rapid Industrialization* (Seattle, WA, 1988), p. 6.

38 Doo-sub Kim and Cheong-seok Kim, *The Population of Korea* (Taejeon, 2004), p. 333.

39 Brandt, *A Korean Village*, pp. 49–51; Dennis Hart, *From Tradition to Consumption: Construction of a Capitalist Culture in South Korea* (Seoul, 2001), pp. 27, 42–3.

40 Andrei Lankov, *The Dawn of Modern Korea: The Transformation in Life and Cityscape* (Seoul, 2007), pp. 166–7.

41 Command of Major General Brown (signed by Colonel, AGD, Adjutant General Charles Ennis), Letter HQ XXIV Corps, APO 235, Office of the Commanding General, TFYQM 430, to Chief Seoul Billeting Section APO 235, dated 31 March 1947, Subj.: Mess Inspection Supper Meal 24 March 47 and Breakfast Meal 25 March 47. U.S. National Archives NARA Archives. Record Group 554, Box 98, Folder: Subsistence Stores 1947.

42 Young-kyun Yang, 'Jajangmyeon and Junggukjip: The Changing Position and Meaning of Chinese Food and Chinese Restaurants in Korean Society', *Korea Journal*, XLV/2 (2005), pp. 64, 71. See also *Chosŏn Ilbo*, 2 December 1971, after Park, 'Kankoku oyobi Nihon ni okeru', pp. 33–4.

43 Lotte 'Company Profile' and 'About Lotte', at www.lotte.co.jp (accessed 15 September 2010).

44 Korean Nutrition Society, *Korean Nutrition Resource Data*, p. 121. See also Andrei Lankov, 'Experience to Go', *Korea Times*, 25 October 2007, at www.koreatimes.co.kr (accessed 15 September 2010).

45 Jaechul Jung and Hun-hee Kim, 'American Fast Food Industry in Korea', research paper 903M16. Ivey School of Business, University of Western Ontario (2003), p. 13.

46 Observations based on author's fieldwork in central Seoul, September–December 2003.
47 Nelson, *Measured Excess*, p. 70.
48 Sangmee Bak, 'McDonald's in Seoul: Food Choices, Identity, and Nationalism', in *Golden Arches East: McDonald's in East Asia*, ed. James L. Watson (Stanford, CA, 1997), pp. 150, 154.
49 Sangmee Bak, 'Negotiating National and Transnational Identities through Consumption Choices: Hamburgers, Espresso, and Mobile Technologies among Koreans', *Review of Korean Studies*, VII/2 (2004), pp. 35–6; and Suk Lee, 'Food Shortage and Economic Institutions in the Democratic People's Republic of Korea', PhD dissertation, University of Warwick (2003), pp. 141–2, 238, available at http://wrap.warwick.ac.uk (accessed 2 September 2011).
50 Park, 'Kankoku oyobi Nihon ni okeru', pp. 117–18.
51 Michael J. Pettid, *Korean Cuisine: An Illustrated History* (London, 2008), pp. 59–62.
52 Boudewijn C. A. Walraven, 'Bardot Soup and Confucians' Meat: Food and Korean Identity in Global Context', in *Asian Food: The Global and the Local*, ed. K. J. Cwiertka with B.C.A. Walraven (Honolulu, HI, 2002), pp. 102–3; Sorensen, *Over the Mountains Are Mountains*, pp. 111–18.
53 Sorensen, *Over the Mountains Are Mountains*, p. 95.
54 Andrew F. Smith, *The Oxford Companion to American Food and Drink* (Oxford, 2007), p. 559. See also Carolyn Wyman, *Spam: A Biography* (San Diego, New York, London, 1999).
55 Sumiko Kaneshiro, 'Okinawa no shokuseikatsu ni miru Amerika tōji no eikyō', in *Sengo Okinawa to Amerika: Ibunka sesshoku no 50 nen*, ed. Teruya Yoshihiko and Yamazato Katsunori (Naha, 1995), pp. 160–64; Ty Matejowsky, 'SPAM and Fast-food "Glocalization" in the Philippines', *Food, Culture and Society*, X/1 (2007), p. 26.
56 Helen-Louise Brown, 'Conceived in the Past and Raised in Modernity: A Study of the Korean Barbecue Restaurant', MA dissertation, University of Adelaide (2010), p. 14.
57 Ibid., pp. 23–5, 30.
58 Ibid., p. 28.
59 Ibid., p. 42.
60 Renee B. Kim, 'Meeting Consumer Concerns for Food Safety in South Korea: The Importance of Food Safety and Ethics in a Globalizing Market', *Journal of Agricultural and Environmental Ethics*, XXII/2 (2009), p. 142.

61 Brown, 'Conceived in the Past and Raised in Modernity', p. 56.

62 Robert W. Pemberton, 'Wild-gathered Foods as Countercurrents to Dietary Globalisation in South Korea', in *Asian Food: The Global and the Local*, ed. Cwiertka with Walraven, pp. 79–80.

63 Nelson, *Measured Excess*, pp. 126–30.

64 Laura C. Nelson, 'South Korean Consumer Nationalism: Women, Children, Credit, and Other Perils', in *The Ambivalent Consumer: Questioning Consumption in East Asia and the West*, ed. S. Garon and P. L. Maclachlan (Ithaca, NY, 2006), p. 192.

65 Ibid., p. 195.

66 Ibid., p. 205.

67 Sangmee Bak, 'Exoticizing the Familiar, Domesticating the Foreign: Ethnic Food Restaurants in Korea', *Korea Journal*, L/1 (2010), pp. 110–32; Bak, 'Negotiating National and Transnational Identities', pp. 37–42.

68 For example, Susan J. Terrio, 'Crafting *Grand Cru* Chocolates in Contemporary France', in *The Cultural Politics of Food and Eating: A Reader*, ed. J. L. Watson and M. L. Caldwell (New York and London, 2005).

69 Han'guk oesik chŏngbo, *Han'guk oesik yŏn'gam*, p. 314.

70 Nelson, *Measured Excess*, p. 25.

71 Dennis L. McNamara, *The Colonial Origins of Korean Enterprise, 1910–1945* (Cambridge, MA, 1990), p. 127.

72 Ibid., pp. 130–32.

73 Bureau of Statistics, Ministry of Home Affairs, ed., *Statistical Yearbook of the Republic of Korea, 1957* (Seoul, 1957), p. 104.

74 Han'guk unheng chosabu, ed., *Kyŏngje yŏn'gam* (Seoul, 1956), p. 103.

75 Ministry of Health and Social Affairs, ed., *Year Book of Public Health and Social Statistics, 1961* (Seoul, 1962), p. 178.

76 Kyŏngje kiwŏn, ed., *Kyŏngje paekji* (Seoul, 1962), pp. 82–4.

77 Korean Nutrition Society, *Korean Nutrition Resource Data*, pp. 274–5.

78 See, for example, *Chosŏn Ilbo*, 9 July 1965, p. 2; 12 May 1966, p. 2; 24 July 1966, p. 5; 20 September 1966, p. 8; 23 December 1966, p. 1.

79 Kyung-koo Han, 'The "Kimchi Wars" in Globalizing East Asia: Consuming Class, Gender, Health, and National Identity', in *Consuming Korean Tradition in Early and Late Modernity*, ed. L. Kendall (Honolulu, HI, 2010), pp. 141–2.

80 Chong Dae Sung, *Yakiniku, kimuchi to Nihonjin* (Tokyo, 2004), pp. 127, 135.

81 'Japan Korea Kimchi Dispute', TED case studies, at www1.american.edu (accessed 22 April 2011).

82 Han, 'The "Kimchi Wars"', p. 143.

83 Theodore Jun Yoo, 'Shaken or Stirred? Taking Something Plebian to Wash Down All That "Hansik": Recreating Makgŏlli for the 21st Century'. Paper presented at the annual meeting of the Association for Asian Studies, Honolulu, HI, March–April 2011.

84 'Makgeolli Exports to Japan Exceed Sake Imports', *The Chosun Ilbo*, 27 January 2012, at http://english.chosun.com (accessed 14 August 2012).

85 Okpyo Moon, 'Food and Food Consumption as Cultural Practices: Lifestyle Changes in Contemporary Korea?', *Korea Journal*, L/1 (2010), p. 7.

86 Zygmunt Bauman, *Consuming Life* (Cambridge, 2007).

87 Theodore C. Bestor, *Tsukiji: The Fish Market at the Center of the World* (Berkeley, CA, 2004), pp. 146–7, 159–60; Sea-Ling Cheng, 'Back to the Future: Herbal Tea Shops in Hong Kong', in *Hong Kong: The Anthropology of a Chinese Metropolis*, ed. G. Evans and M. Tam (Richmond, Surrey, 1997), pp. 51–73; Yunxiang Yan, 'Of Hamburger and Social Space: Consuming McDonald's in Beijing', in *The Cultural Politics of Food and Eating: A Reader*, ed. J. L. Watson and M. L. Caldwell (Malden and Oxford, 2005), pp. 80–103.

88 Laurel Kendall, 'Introduction: Material Modernity, Consumable Tradition', in *Consuming Korean Tradition in Early and Late Modernity: Commodification, Tourism and Performance*, ed. L. Kendall (Honolulu, HI, 2010), p. 3.

89 For details on the Royal Palace cuisine see Pettid, *Korean Cuisine*, pp. 128–41.

90 Keith Howard, *Bands, Songs, and Shamanistic Rituals: Folk Music in Korean Society* (Seoul, 1989), p. 242.

91 Roald Maliangkay, 'Choosing the Right Folk: The Appointment of "Human Cultural Properties" in Korea', in *Folksong: Tradition, Revival, and Re-creation*, ed. I. Russell and D. Atkinson (Aberdeen, 2004), p. 96.

92 Okpyo Moon, 'Dining Elegance and Authenticity: Archaeology of Royal Court Cuisine in Korea', in *Korea Journal*, L/1 (2010), pp. 45–8.

93 See www.jihwajafood.co.kr (accessed 2 September 2011).

94 Observations based on author's fieldwork in central Seoul, September–December 2003. See also Katarzyna J. Cwiertka, 'Daejanggeum and the Gentrification of Korean Food Culture', *Korea Foundation Newsletter*, XIII/1 (2004), at http://newsletter.kf.or.kr (accessed 2 September 2011).

95 See, for example, *Yang-mi Kyŏng kwa hamkke hanŭn 'Taejanggŭm suragan kungjugn yori'* (MBC DVD set, 2004) and Han Pong-nyŏ, *Chip esŏ mandŭnŭn kungjung ŭmsik* (Seoul, 2004). For more information about

the institute see www.food.co.kr (accessed 30 September 2010).

96 Moon, 'Dining Elegance and Authenticity', pp. 48–9.

6 North Korea's Bumpy Road to Affluence

1 'NK's First Fast Food Outlet Enjoying Popularity', 12 October 2009, at www.koreatimes.co.kr; Bernice Han, '"Minced Beef and Bread" at NKorean Fast Food Joint', 11 October 2009, at www.thejakartaglobe.com; Bernice Han, '"Minced Beef and Bread" a Hit in North Korean Fast Food Joint', 12 October 2009, at www.chinapost.com.tw (all accessed 10 August 2011).

2 James L. Watson, *Golden Arches East: McDonald's in East Asia* (Stanford, CA, 1997); Yan Yunxiang, 'Of Hamburger and Social Space: Consuming McDonald's in Beijing', in *The Cultural Politics of Food and Eating: A Reader*, ed. James L. Watson and M. Caldwell (New York, 2005).

3 'Samtaesong Fast Food Restaurant in Pyongyang', North Korean Economy Watch, at www.nkeconwatch.com (accessed 10 August 2011).

4 See 'Waffletown', on the blog www.ladyironchef.com, 2 July 2008, for more details on the Singapore Waffletown outlets (accessed 10 December 2009).

5 Jukka Gronow, *Caviar with Champagne: Common Luxury and the Ideals of the Good Life in Stalin's Russia* (Oxford, 2004), pp. 73–4.

6 Andrei Lankov, *North of the DMZ: Essays on Daily Life in North Korea* (Jefferson, NC, 2007), p. 93.

7 NK Brief No. 08-7-4-1, posted on 4 July 2008, at http://ifes.kyungnam.ac.kr (accessed 10 August 2009).

8 Barbara Demick, *Nothing to Envy: Real Lives in North Korea* (London, 2010), pp. 75, 136.

9 Ibid., pp. 150–51. For more accounts on the North Korean markets see pp. 154–7.

10 NK Brief No. 09-3-26-1, at http://ifes.kyungnam.ac.kr (accessed 10 December 2009). Currently no longer available online.

11 Robert Willoughby, *North Korea: The Bradt Travel Guide* (Chalfont St Peter, Bucks, 2008), p. 108.

12 Rob Whyte, *Korea* (Lonely Planet Country Guide) (n.p., 2007), p. 367.

13 'Pizza Parlor opens in Pyongyang, DPRK', and 'N. Korea's First Fast Food Joint', at www.youtube.com (accessed 30 August 2010). For images of fast food, pizza and pasta served in restaurants in Pyongyang see also the slide show on Leonid Petrov's site, 'Fast Food Becomes

Popular in Pyongyang', at http://leonidpetrov.wordpress.com (accessed 10 December 2009).

14 Lankov, *North of the DMZ*, p. 90.

15 The ad is available on YouTube as 'KCTV (Quail Restaurant in Pyongyang)', www.youtube.com (accessed 27 November 2009).

16 Jon Herskovitz, 'North Korean Beer: Great Taste, Low Proliferation Risk', Reuters Canada, 9 March 2008, at http://ca.reuters.com (accessed 12 December 2009).

17 To view the beer advert see 'Taedonggang Beer (North Korean beer commercial)', at www.youtube.com; for an English commentary see 'North Korea Promotes "Healthy" Beer', at www.youtube.com (accessed 30 August 2010).

18 'N. Korean Leader Pulls Plug on TV Commercials: Sources', *Yonhap News*, 8 November 2008, at http://english.yonhapnews.co.kr (accessed 10 December 2009).

19 See Andrew S. Natsios, *The Great North Korean Famine* (Washington, DC, 2001), p. 6.

20 Suk Lee, 'Food Shortages and Economic Institutions in the Democratic People's Republic of Korea', PhD dissertation, University of Warwick (2003), p. 168, available at http://wrap.warwick.ac.uk (accessed 2 September 2011).

21 Paul French, *North Korea: The Paranoid Peninsula – A Modern History* (London, 2004), p. 130.

22 Lee, 'Food Shortages and Economic Institutions', p. 219; Hazel Smith, *Hungry for Peace: International Security, Humanitarian Assistance and Social Change in North Korea* (Washington, DC, 2005), pp. 73, 252–3; Stephan Haggard and Marcus Noland, *Famine in North Korea: Markets, Aid and Reform* (New York, 2007), p.1.

23 Haggard and Noland, *Famine in North Korea*, p. 7.

24 Ibid., pp. 91–2.

25 Sunyoung Pak, 'The Growth Status of North Korean Refugee Children in China', *Korea Journal*, XLIII/3 (2003), p. 179.

26 National Intelligence Council, *Strategic Implications of Global Health* (2008), p. 6; 'Special Products' section, at www.dni.gov (accessed 13 January 2010).

27 Pak, 'The Growth Status of North Korean Refugee Children', p. 172.

28 Daniel Schwekendiek, 'The North Korean Standard of Living during the Famine', *Social Science and Medicine*, 66 (2008), p. 597.

29 Pak, 'The Growth Status of North Korean Refugee Children', p. 175. For details of the nutritional survey conducted in North Korea see World

Food Programme, *Full Report of the Evaluation of DPRK EMOPs 5959.00 & 5959.01* (Rome, 2000), at www.wfp.org (accessed 1 February 2010).

30 Pak, 'The Growth Status of North Korean Refugee Children', p. 166.

31 Haggard and Noland, *Famine in North Korea*, p. 81.

32 Smith, *Hungry for Peace*, pp. 108–9.

33 Ibid., pp. 106–8.

34 World Food Programme (WFP) DPR Korea Country Office, LFP Unit, *Report on Local Food Production Factories containing WFP Equipment, December 2007–January 2008* (Rome, 2008).

35 WFP Strategy and Policy Division, Technical Unit (Nutrition), *Fortified Blended Foods: Recipes, Facts and Practical Uses* (Rome, 2002), pp. 18–19, 26.

36 WFP Executive Board Documents, Protracted Relief and Recovery Operation – Democratic People's Republic of Korea 10488.0, p. 3.

37 Food and Agriculture Organization/World Food Programme, *Special Report: FAO/WFP Crop and Food Security Assessment Mission to the Democratic People's Republic of Korea, November 2008* (Rome, 2008), p. 22. See also World Food Programme, *10757.0 – Emergency Assistance to Population Groups Affected by Floods and Rising Food and Fuel Prices* (Rome, 2008). Electronic document, at www.wfp.org (accessed 30 August 2010, no longer available at this URL).

38 See Natsios, *The Great North Korean Famine*, and Haggard and Noland, *Famine in North Korea*. Both books offer an extensive bibliography for further exploration.

39 Natsios, *The Great North Korean Famine*, pp. 14–16; Haggard and Noland, *Famine in North Korea*, p. 26.

40 Haggard and Noland, *Famine in North Korea*, pp. 3, 9.

41 Lee, 'Food Shortages and Economic Institutions', p. 220.

42 Mun Woong Lee, 'Rural North Korea under Communism: A Study of Sociocultural Change', PhD dissertation, Rice University, Houston (1975), pp. 25–7.

43 Lee, 'Food Shortages and Economic Institutions', pp. 115–17. See also Lee, 'Rural North Korea', pp. 68–77.

44 Lee, 'Food Shortages and Economic Institutions', pp. 15–8, 73–4.

45 A Korean unit of land measurement. One *chŏngbo* translates to approximately 2.45 acres or 0.99 hectares.

46 Lee, 'Rural North Korea', pp. 54–67.

47 Lee, 'Food Shortages and Economic Institutions', pp. 10, 30.

48 Keith Pratt and Richard Rutt, *Korea: A Historical and Cultural Dictionary* (Richmond, Surrey, 1999), p. 67. See also Michael E. Robinson, *Korea's*

Twentieth-Century Odyssey: A Short History (Honolulu, HI, 2007), pp. 158–6[illegible] and French, *North Korea*, pp. 30–47.

49 Lee, 'Food Shortages and Economic Institutions', p. 130.

50 Ibid., p. 148.

51 Lee, 'Rural North Korea', p. 73.

52 Lee, 'Food Shortages and Economic Institutions', pp. 12–13. ee also Haggard and Noland, *Famine in North Korea*, pp. 24–7.

53 Lee, 'Food Shortages and Economic Institutions', pp. 162–4.

54 Ibid., pp. 29, 58–9, 71–2.

55 Ibid., pp. 97–8.

56 Helen-Louise Hunter, *Kim Il-song's North Korea* (Westport, CT, and London, 1999), p. 162.

57 Lee, 'Food Shortages and Economic Institutions', pp. 141–2. See also p. 238.

58 Ibid., pp. 201, 218, 232, 255–6.

59 Ibid., pp. 21–2, 99–101.

60 French, *North Korea*, pp. 119, 130.

61 Charles K. Armstrong, *The North Korean Revolution, 1945–1950* (Ithaca, NY, 2003), p. 144.

62 Lankov, *North of the DMZ*, p. 229; Hunter, *Kim Il-song's North Korea*, pp. 162–3; Ralph Hassig and Kongdan Oh, *The Hidden People of North Korea: Everyday Life in the Hermit Kingdom* (Lanham, MD, 2009), p. 113.

63 Hunter, *Kim Il-song's North Kore*a, p. 154.

64 Demick, *Nothing to Envy*, p. 68.

65 Lankov, *North of the DMZ*, p. 230.

66 World Food Programme, *Full Report of the Evaluation of DPRK EMOPs*, p. 16.

67 Lankov, *North of the DMZ*, pp. 228–30.

68 Yi Ki-ch'un et al., *T'ongil e ap'sŏ ponŭn Pukhan ŭi kajŏng saenghwal munhwa* (Seoul, 2001), pp. 194–6.

69 Lee, 'Food Shortages and Economic Institutions', pp. 25–6, 30, 89.

70 Ibid., p. 103.

71 Ibid., pp. 141–2, 293–4.

72 Ibid., pp. 141–2.

73 Ibid., p. 295.

74 Lankov, *North of the DMZ*, p. 316.

75 Lee, 'Food Shortages and Economic Institutions', p. 296. See also Lankov, *North of the DMZ*, p. 318.

76 Lankov, *North of the DMZ*, p. 318.

77 Ibid., pp. 317–18. For an extensive account of North Korean markets

see Demick, *Nothing to Envy*, pp. 154–7.

78 FAO/WFP, *Special Report*, p. 26.

79 Ibid., p. 24.

80 Lee, 'Food Shortages and Economic Institutions', pp. 280–81.

81 French, *North Korea*, pp. 140–41.

82 Sheila Fitzpatrick, *Everyday Stalinism. Ordinary Life in Extraordinary Times: Soviet Russia in the 1930s* (Oxford, 1999), pp. 95–109. See also Jukka Gronow, *Caviar with Champagne: Common Luxury and the Ideals of the Good Life in Stalin's Russia* (Oxford, 2004).

83 Hunter, *Kim Il-song's North Korea*, pp. 130, 141, 144.

84 Sunyoung Pak, 'The Biological Standard of Living in the Two Koreas', *Economics and Human Biology*, 2 (2004), p. 520.

85 Pak, 'The Biological Standard of Living', p. 512.

86 Daniel Schwekendiek and Sunyoung Pak, 'Recent Growth of Children in the Two Koreas: A Meta-analysis', *Economics and Human Biology*, 7 (2009), pp. 109–12.

87 Armstrong, *The North Korean Revolution*, p. 4.

88 David Heather and Koen de Ceuster, *North Korean Posters* (Munich, 2008), pp. 15, 22–4, 26–30, 32–3, 39–42, 56–8.

89 Hunter, *Kim Il-song's North Korea*, p. 112.

90 Yi et al., *T'ongil e ap'sŏ ponŭn Pukhan ŭi kajŏng saengwhal munhwa*, pp. 200–2.

91 Ibid., pp. 181–2; Michael J. Pettid, *Korean Cuisine: An Illustrated History* (London, 2008), pp. 52–3, 104. See also Clark W. Sorensen, *Over the Mountains Are Mountains: Korean Peasant Households and Their Adaptations to Rapid Industrialization* (Seattle, WA, 1988), pp. 91–118.

92 FAO, *Special Report*, pp. 23, 25.

93 Yi et al., *T'ongil e ap'sŏ ponŭn Pukhan ŭi kajŏng saengwhal munhwa*, p. 183.

94 Lankov, *North of the DMZ*, pp. 215–16.

95 Hunter, *Kim Il-song's North Korea*, p. 164.

96 Sorensen, *Over the Mountains Are Mountains*, p. 100.

Conclusion

1 Sidney W. Mintz, *Sweetness and Power: The Place of Sugar in Modern History* (New York, 1985); Helen Macbeth, ed., *Food Preferences and Taste: Continuity and Change* (Providence, RI, and Oxford, 1997); Paul Rozin, *Towards a Psychology of Food Choice* (Brussels, 1998); Marianne

E. Lien and Brigitte Nerlich, eds, *The Politics of Food* (Oxford and New York, 2004); James L. Watson and Melissa L. Caldwell, eds, *The Cultural Politics of Food and Eating: A Reader* (New York, 2005).

2 Dennis L. McNamara, *The Colonial Origins of Korean Enterprise, 1910–1945* (Cambridge, New York and Melbourne, 1990); Carter J. Eckert, *Offsprings of Empire: The Koch'ang Kims and the Colonial Origins of Korean Capitalism, 1876–1945* (Seattle, WA, 1991).

3 Sidney W. Mintz, *Tasting Food, Tasting Freedom: Excursions into Eating, Culture, and the Past* (Boston, MA, 1996), p. 25.

4 Roy Richard Grinker, *Korea and Its Futures: Unification and the Unfinished War* (New York, 1998), pp. 8–10.

5 Ibid., p. 8.

6 Ibid., pp. 7–8.

7 Laurel Kendall, 'Introduction: Material Modernity, Consumable Tradition', in *Consuming Korean Tradition in Early and Late Modernity: Commodification, Tourism and Performance*, ed. L. Kendall (Honolulu, HI, 2010), p. 6.

Tables and Charts

1 Michael E. Robinson, *Korea's Twentieth-Century Odyssey: A Short History* (Honolulu, HI, 2007), p. 38.

2 Keijō kankō kyōkai, *Keijō kankō annai zu* (Keijō, 1934), back cover.

3 Tsushima, 'Chōsen ni okeru miso oyobi shōyu jōzō no genjō ni tsuite', *Shokugin Chōsa Geppō*, 61 (1943), p. 12.

4 Taehan changnyu kong'ŏp hyŏptong chohap, ed., *Taehan changnyu kong'ŏp hyŏptong chohap 35 nyŏn sa* (Seoul, 1997), pp. 81–3.

5 Bruce F. Johnston with Mosaburo Hosoda and Yoshio Kusumi, *Japanese Food Management in World War II* (Stanford, CA, 1953), p. 203.

6 Kyoung-hee Park, 'Food Rationing and the Black Market in Wartime Korea', in *Food and War in Mid-Twentieth-Century East Asia*, ed. K. J. Cwiertka (Farnham, forthcoming).

7 Data based on Government food rationing decrees, after Suk Lee, 'Food Shortages and Economic Institutions in the Democratic People's Republic of Korea', PhD dissertation, University of Warwick (2003), p. 61. Available at http://wrap.warwick.ac.uk (accessed 2 September 2011).

8 After Young-kyun Yang, 'Jajangmyeon and Junggukjip: The Changing Position and Meaning of Chinese Food and Chinese Restaurants in

Korean Society', *Korea Journal*, XLV/2 (2005), p. 71.

9 Han'guk oesik chŏngbo, *Han'guk oesik yŏn'gam* (Seoul, 2009), p. 314.

10 Based on the fieldwork conducted by the author in central Seoul, September–December 2003.

11 The Korean Nutrition Society, *Korean Nutrition Resource Data* (Seoul, 1989), p. 276.

12 Lee, 'Food Shortages and Economic Insitutions', p. 149.

13 Ibid., p. 249.

14 Ajinomoto kabushiki kaisha, ed., *Ajinomoto enkakushi* (Tokyo, 1951), pp. 798–9.

15 Tsushima, 'Chōsen ni okeru miso oyobi shōyu', p. 13.

16 Cohen, *Japan's Economy in War and Reconstruction* (Minneapolis, MN, 1949), p. 369. The crop year does not correspond with the calendar year, but lasts from 1 November to 31 October.

17 Keijō shōkō kaigisho, ed., *Chōsen ni okeru busshi no haikyū tōsei to haikyū kikō* (Keijō, 1943), p. 42.

18 Mun Woong Lee, 'Rural North Korea Under Communism: A Study of Socio-cultural Change', PhD dissertation, Rice University, Houston, Texas (1975), p. 60.

Select Bibliography

Ahn, Junghyo, *Silver Stallion: A Novel of Korea* (New York, 1990)

Armstrong, Charles K., *The North Korean Revolution, 1945–1950* (Ithaca, NY, 2003)

Bak, Sangmee, 'McDonald's in Seoul: Food Choices, Identity, and Nationalism', in *Golden Arches East: McDonald's in East Asia*, ed. James L. Watson (Stanford, CA, 1997), pp. 136–60

—, 'Negotiating National and Transnational Identities through Consumption Choices: Hamburgers, Espresso, and Mobile Technologies among Koreans', *Review of Korean Studies*, VII/2 (2004), pp. 33–52

—, 'Exoticizing the Familiar, Domesticating the Foreign: Ethnic Food Restaurants in Korea', *Korea Journal*, L/1 (2010), pp. 110–32

Baldwin, Coy W., 'Food Service United Nations', *The Quartermaster Review*, XXXII/6 (1953), pp. 20–21, 116–17

Brandt, Vincent S. R., *A Korean Village: Between Farm and Sea* (Cambridge, MA, 1971)

Brazinsky, Gregg, *Nation Building in South Korea: Koreans, Americans, and the Making of Democracy* (Chapel Hill, NC, 2007)

Breuker, Remco, 'Korea's Forgotten War: Appropriating and Subverting the Vietnam War in Korean Popular Imaginings', *Korean Histories*, I/1 (2009), pp. 36–59

Brown, Helen-Louise, 'Conceived in the Past and Raised in Modernity: A Study of the Korean Barbecue Restaurant', MA thesis, University of Adelaide (2010)

Brune, Lester H., ed., *The Korean War: Handbook of the Literature and Research* (Westport, CT, 1996)

Bureau of Statistics, Ministry of Home Affairs, ed., *Statistical Yearbook of the Republic of Korea, 1957* (Seoul, 1957)

Burmeister, Larry L., 'Agricultural Cooperative Development and Change: A Window on South Korea's Agrarian Transformation', in *Transformations in Twentieth-Century Korea*, ed. Chang Yun-shik and Steven Hugh Lee (London, 2006), pp. 64–86
Chae, Kyung Oh, *The Handbook of Korea* (New York, 1958)
Ch'ae, Man-sik, 'A Ready-made Life' [1934], trans. Chong-un Kim and Bruce Dulton, in *A Ready-made Life: Early Masters of Modern Korean Fiction* (Honolulu, HI, 1998)
Chang, Yunshik, 'Colonization as Planned Change: The Korean Case', *Modern Asian Studies*, V/2 (1971), pp. 161–86
Choi, Hochin, 'The Strengthening of the Economic Domination by Japanese Colonialism (1932–1945): Statistical Analysis', *Yŏnsei Nonch'ong*, 7 (1969), pp. 349–78
Chu, Young-Ha, 'Origin and Change in *Kimch'i* Culture', *Korea Journal*, XXXV/2 (1995), pp. 18–29
Chung, Donald K., *The Three Day Promise: A Korean Soldier's Memoir* (Tallahassee, FL, 1989)
Cohen, Nicole, 'Children of Empire: Growing up Japanese in Colonial Korea, 1876–1946', PhD dissertation, Columbia University, New York (2006)
Conway-Lanz, Sahr, 'Beyond No Gun Ri: Refugees and the United States Military in the Korean War', *Diplomatic History*, XXIX/1 (2005), pp. 49–81
Cumings, Bruce, *The Origins of the Korean War*, vol. I: *Liberation and the Emergence of Separate Regimes, 1945–1947* (Princeton, NJ, 1981)
—, *The Origins of the Korean War*, vol. II: *The Roaring of the Cataract, 1947–1950* (Princeton, NJ, 1990)
—, *The Korean War: A History* (New York, 2010)
—, 'The Legacy of Japanese Colonialism in Korea', in *The Japanese Colonial Empire, 1895–1945*, ed. R. H. Myers and M. R. Peattie (Princeton, NJ, 1984), pp. 478–96
Cwiertka, Katarzyna J., *Modern Japanese Cuisine: Food, Power and National Identity* (London, 2006)
—, 'Daejanggeum and the Gentrification of Korean Food Culture', *Korea Foundation Newsletter*, XIII/1 (2004)
—, ed. *Food and War in Mid-Twentieth-Century East Asia* (Farnham, forthcoming)
—, and Akiko Moriya, 'Fermented Soyfoods in South Korea: The Industrialization of Tradition', in *The World of Soy*, ed. C. Du Bois, C. B. Tan and S. Mintz (Urbana, IL, 2008), pp. 161–81

Delissen, Alain, 'Denied and Besieged: The Japanese of Korea, 1876–1945', in *New Frontiers: Imperialism's New Communities in East Asia, 1842–1953*, ed. R. Bickers and C. Henriot (Manchester, 2000), pp. 125–45

Demick, Barbara, *Nothing to Envy: Real Lives in North Korea* (London, 2010)

Dowdey, Patrick, ed., *Living Through the Forgotten War: Portrait of Korea* (Middletown, CT, 2004)

Duus, Peter, *The Abacus and the Sword: The Japanese Penetration of Korea, 1895–1910* (Berkeley, CA, 1995)

Eckert, Carter, *Offsprings of Empire: The Koch'ang Kims and the Colonial Origins of Korean Capitalism, 1876–1945* (Seattle, WA, 1991)

—, 'Total War, Industrialization, and Social Change in Late Colonial Korea', in *The Japanese Wartime Empire, 1931–1945*, ed. P. Duus, R. H. Myers and M. R. Peattie (Princeton, NJ, 1996), pp. 3–39

—, et al., *Korea Old and New: A History* (Seoul, 1990)

Francks, Penelope, 'Rice for the Masses: Food Policy and the Adoption of Imperial Self-sufficiency in Early Twentieth-century Japan', *Japan Forum*, XV/1 (2003), pp. 125–46

French, Paul, *North Korea: The Paranoid Peninsula – A Modern History* (London, 2004)

Grajdanzev, Andrew J., *Modern Korea* (New York, 1944)

Grinker, Roy Richard, *Korea and Its Futures: Unification and the Unfinished War* (New York, 1998)

Haggard, Stephan, and Marcus Noland, *Famine in North Korea: Markets, Aid and Reform* (New York, 2007)

Hahm, Hanhee, 'Rice and Koreans: Three Identities and Meanings', *Korea Journal*, XLV/2 (2005), pp. 89–106

Han, Kyung-koo, 'The "Kimchi Wars" in Globalizing East Asia: Consuming Class, Gender, Health, and National Identity', in *Consuming Korean Tradition in Early and Late Modernity*, ed. L. Kendall (Honolulu, HI, 2010), pp. 21–38

Hassig, Ralph, and Kongdan Oh, *The Hidden People of North Korea: Everyday Life in the Hermit Kingdom* (Lanham, MD, 2009)

Hayami, Yujiro, and Vernon W. Ruttan, 'Korean Rice, Taiwan Rice, and Japanese Agricultural Stagnation: An Economic Consequence of Colonialism', *The Quarterly Journal of Economics*, LXXXIV/4 (1970), pp. 562–89

Heather, David, and Koen de Ceuster, *North Korean Posters* (Munich, 2008)

Henry, Todd Andrew, 'Keijō: Japanese and Korean Constructions of Colonial Seoul and the History of Its Lived Spaces, 1910–1945', PhD dissertation, University of California (2006)

Hepinstall, Hi Soo Shin, *Growing Up in the Korean Kitchen: A Cookbook* (Berkeley, CA, 2001)
Ho, Samuel Pao-San, 'Colonialism and Development: Korea, Taiwan and Kwantung', in *The Japanese Colonial Empire, 1895–1945*, ed. R. H. Myers and M. R. Peattie (Princeton, NJ, 1984), pp. 347–98
Hunter, Helen-Louise, *Kim Il-song's North Korea* (Westport, CT, and London, 1999)
Huston, James A., *Guns and Butter, Powder and Rice: U.S. Army Logistics in the Korean War* (London and Toronto, 1989)
Hwang, Sunwŏn, trans. Bruce and Ju-chan Fulton, 'The Toad', in *Lost Souls: Stories* (New York, 2010), pp. 158–85
Jacobson, Mark R., '"Minds Then Hearts": U.S. Political and Psychological Warfare During the Korean War', PhD dissertation, Ohio State University (2005)
Johnston, Bruce F., Mosaburo Hosoda and Yoshio Kusumi, *Japanese Food Management in World War II* (Stanford, CA, 1953)
Jung, Jaechul, and Hun-hee Kim, 'American Fast Food Industry in Korea', research paper 903M16. Ivey School of Business, University of Western Ontario (2003)
Jung, Keun-sik, 'Colonial Modernity and the Social History of Chemical Seasoning in Korea', *Korea Journal*, XLV/2 (2005), pp. 9–36
Kendall, Laurel, 'Introduction: Material Modernity, Consumable Tradition', in *Consuming Korean Tradition in Early and Late Modernity: Commodification, Tourism and Performance*, ed. L. Kendall (Honolulu, HI, 2010), pp. 1–18
Kim, Doo-sub, and Cheong-seok Kim, *The Population of Korea* (Taejeon, 2004)
Kim, Janice C. H., *To Live to Work: Factory Women in Colonial Korea, 1910–1945* (Stanford, CA, 2009)
Kim, Kirk Y. K., 'The Impact of Japanese Colonial Development on the Korean Economy', *Korea Journal*, XVII/1 (1977), pp. 12–21
Kim, Kwang-ok, 'Contested Terrain of Imagination: Chinese Food in Korea', in *Changing Chinese Foodways in Asia*, ed. D.Y.H. Wu and C. B. Tan (Hong Kong, 2001), pp. 201–17
—, 'Rice Cuisine and Cultural Practice in Contemporary Korean Dietary Life', *Korea Journal*, L/1 (2010), pp. 11–34
Kim, Renee B., 'Meeting Consumer Concerns for Food Safety in South Korea: The Importance of Food Safety and Ethics in a Globalizing Market', *Journal of Agricultural and Environmental Ethics*, XXII/2 (2009), pp. 141–52

The Korean Nutrition Society, *Korean Nutrition Resources Data* (Seoul, 1989)
The Korean Reconstruction Bank, ed., *Industry in Korea: 1967* (Seoul, 1967)
Kuznets, Paul W., 'Causes, Consequences, Relevance: Korea's Industrialization', in *Transformations in Twentieth-Century Korea*, ed. Chang Yun-shik and Steven Hugh Lee (London, 2006), pp. 89–105
Lankov, Andrei, *The Dawn of Modern Korea: The Transformation in Life and Cityscape* (Seoul, 2007)
—, *North of the DMZ: Essays on Daily Life in North Korea* (Jefferson, NC, 2007)
Lee, Helie, *Still Life with Rice: A Young American Woman Discovers the Life and Legacy of Her Korean Grandmother* (New York, 1996)
Lee, Jong-Won, 'The Impact of the Korean War on the Korean Economy', *International Journal of Korean Studies*, v/1 (2001), pp. 97–118
Lee, Mun Woong, 'Rural North Korea Under Communism: A Study of Socio-cultural Change', PhD dissertation, Rice University, Houston, Texas (1975)
Lee, Seung-nam, 'Analytical Study of Influxes of Korean Rice and the Korean Rice Production Development Program: 1910–1939', *Hokkaidō Daigaku Nōkei Ronsō*, 40 (1984), pp. 175–98
Lee, Suk, 'Food Shortages and Economic Institutions in the Democratic People's Republic of Korea', PhD dissertation, University of Warwick (2003), available at http://wrap.warwick.ac.uk
Lyons, Jake, 'Feeding the United Nations in Korea', *The Quartermaster Review*, xxxi/1 (1951), pp. 6–7, 150–52
Maliangkay, Roald, 'Choosing the Right Folk: The Appointment of "Human Cultural Properties" in Korea', in *Folksong: Tradition, Revival, and Re-creation,* ed. I. Russell and D. Atkinson (Aberdeen, 2004), pp. 95–107
McCune, George M., *Korea Today* (Cambridge, MA, 1950)
McNamara, Dennis L., *The Colonial Origins of Korean Enterprise, 1910–1945* (Cambridge, 1990)
—, *Trade and Transformation in Korea, 1876–1945* (Boulder, CO, 1998)
Millet, Allan R., *The War for Korea, 1945–1950: A House Burning* (Lawrence, KS, 2005)
Ministry of Health and Social Affairs, ed., *Year Book of Public Health and Social Statistics, 1961* (Seoul, 1962)
Mizoguchi, Toshiyuki, 'Economic Growth of Korea under the Japanese Occupation: Background of Industrialization of Korea, 1911–1940', *Hitotsubashi Journal of Economics*, xx/1 (1979), pp. 1–19
Moon, Katharine H. S., *Sex among Allies: Military Prostitution in U.S.–Korea Relations* (New York, 1997)

Moon, Okpyo, 'Dining Elegance and Authenticity: Archaeology of Royal Court Cuisine in Korea', in *Korea Journal*, L/1 (2010), pp. 36–59
Moon, Seungsook, *Militarized Modernity and Gendered Citizenship in South Korea* (Durham, NC, 2005)
Morris, Harriett, *The Art of Korean Cooking* (Rutland, VT, and Tokyo, 1959)
Myers, Ramon H., and Saburō Yamada, 'Agricultural Development in the Empire', in *The Japanese Colonial Empire, 1895–1945*, ed. R. H. Myers and M. R. Peattie (Princeton, NJ, 1984), pp. 420–54
The National Academy of Korean Language, ed., *An Illustrated Guide to Korean Culture: 233 Traditional Key Words* (Seoul, 2002)
Natsios, Andrew S., *The Great North Korean Famine* (Washington, DC, 2001)
Nelson, Laura C., *Measured Excess: Status, Gender, and Consumer Nationalism in South Korea* (New York, 2000)
—, 'South Korean Consumer Nationalism: Women, Children, Credit, and Other Perils', in *The Ambivalent Consumer: Questioning Consumption in East Asia and the West*, ed. S. Garon and P. L. Maclachlan (Ithaca, NY, 2006), pp. 188–208
Osgood, Cornelius, *The Koreans and Their Culture* (New York, 1951)
Pai, Hyung-il, 'Travel Guides to the Empire: The Production of Tourist Images in Colonial Korea', in *Consuming Korean Tradition in Early and Late Modernity*, ed. L. Kendall (Honolulu, HI, 2010), pp. 67–88
Pak, Sunyoung, 'The Growth Status of North Korean Refugee Children in China', *Korea Journal*, XLIII/3 (2003), pp. 385–95
—, 'The Biological Standard of Living in the Two Koreas', *Economics and Human Biology*, 2 (2004), pp. 511–18
Pak, Wan-so, trans. Yu Young-nan, *The Naked Tree* (Ithaca, NY, 1995)
Park, Kyoung-hee, 'State and Food in South Korea: Moulding National Diet in Wartime and Beyond', PhD dissertation, Leiden University (2012)
Park, Soon-won, *Colonial Industrialization and Labor in Korea* (Cambridge, MA, 1999)
Park, Wan-suh, trans. Yu Young-nan and Stephen J. Epstein, *Who Ate Up all the Shinga?* (New York, 2009)
Pemberton, Robert W., 'Wild-gathered Foods as Countercurrents to Dietary Globalisation in South Korea', in *Asian Food: The Global and the Local*, ed. K. J. Cwiertka with B.C.A. Walraven (Honolulu, HI, 2002), pp. 76–94
Pettid, Michael J., *Korean Cuisine: An Illustrated History* (London, 2008)
Poole, Janet, 'Colonial Interiors: Modernist Fiction of Korea', PhD dissertation, Columbia University, New York (2004)
Pratt, Keith, and Richard Rutt, *Korea: A Historical and Cultural Dictionary*

(Richmond, Surrey, 1999)
Reinschmidt, Michael, 'Rice in South Korean Life: The Transformation of Agricultural Icons', in *The Art of Rice: Spirit and Sustenance in Asia*, ed. Roy W. Hamilton (Los Angeles, CA, 2003), pp. 509–25
Roberts, J.A.G., *China to Chinatown: Chinese Food in the West* (London, 2002)
Robinson, Michael E., *Korea's Twentieth-Century Odyssey: A Short History* (Honolulu, HI, 2007)
Sand, Jordan, 'A Short History of MSG: Good Science, Bad Science, and Taste Cultures', *Gastronomica*, v/4 (2005), pp. 38–49
Sandler, Stanley, *The Korean War: No Victors, No Vanquished* (London, 1999)
Schwekendiek, Daniel, 'The North Korean Standard of Living during the Famine', *Social Science and Medicine*, 66 (2008), pp. 596–608
—, and Sunyoung Pak, 'Recent Growth of Children in the Two Koreas: A Meta-analysis', *Economics and Human Biology*, 7 (2009), pp. 109–12
Shin, Eui-hang, 'Effects of the Korean War on Social Structures of the Republic of Korea: A Socio-demographic Analysis', *California Sociologist*, 15 (1992), pp. 21–42
Shin, Gi-wook, *Ethnic Nationalism in Korea: Genealogy, Politics, and Legacy* (Stanford, CA, 2006)
—, and Michael Robinson, ed., *Colonial Modernity in Korea* (Cambridge, MA, 1999)
Shrader, Charles R., *Communist Logistics in the Korean War* (Westport, CT, 1995)
Skroch, Ernest J., 'Quartermaster Advisors in Korea', *The Quartermaster Review*, XXXI/2 (1951), pp. 8–9, 118–23.
Smith, Hazel, *Hungry for Peace: International Security, Humanitarian Assistance and Social Change in North Korea* (Washington, DC, 2005)
Sorensen, Clark W., *Over the Mountains Are Mountains: Korean Peasant Households and Their Adaptations to Rapid Industrialization* (Seattle, WA, 1988)
South Korean Interim Government, National Economic Board, *Annual Report USAMGIK Service of Civilian Supply for 1947* (Seoul, 1948)
Stubbs, Richard, *Rethinking Asia's Economic Miracle: The Political Economy of War, Prosperity and Crisis* (New York, 2005)
Terry, T. Phillip, *Terry's Guide to the Japanese Empire* (Boston and New York, 1933)
Uchida, Jun, *Brokers of Empire: Japanese Settler Colonialism in Korea, 1876–1945* (Cambridge, MA, 2011)
United States Department of State, *North Korea: A Study in the Techniques of Takeover* (Washington, DC, 1961)

Walraven, Boudewijn C. A., 'Bardot Soup and Confucians' Meat: Food and Korean Identity in Global Context', in *Asian Food: The Global and the Local*, ed. K. J. Cwiertka with B.C.A. Walraven (Honolulu, HI, 2002), pp. 95–115

Whyte, Rob, *Korea* (Lonely Planet Country Guide) (n.p., 2007)

Williams, Alex N., 'Subsistence Supply in Korea', *The Quartermaster Review*, XXXII/4 (1953), pp. 29–30, 132–3

Williams, Rosalind H., *Dream Worlds: Mass Consumption in Late Nineteenth-Century France* (Berkeley, CA, 1982)

Willoughby, Robert, *North Korea: The Bradt Travel Guide* (Chalfont St Peter, Bucks, 2008)

Wolff, David, 'Bean There: Toward a Soy-based History of Northeast Asia', *The South Atlantic Quarterly*, XCIX/1 (2000), pp. 241–52

Wo[illegible], Jung-en, *Race to the Swift: State and Finance in Korean Industrialization* (New York, 1991)

Yan, Yunxiang, 'Of Hamburger and Social Space: Consuming McDonald's in Beijing', in *The Cultural Politics of Food and Eating: A Reader*, ed. J. L. Watson and M. L. Caldwell (Malden and Oxford, 2005), pp. 80–103

Yang, Young-kyun, '*Jajangmyeon* and *Junggukjip*: The Changing Position and Meaning of Chinese Food and Chinese Restaurants in Korean Society', *Korea Journal*, XLV/2 (2005), pp. 60–88

Yi, Sang, 'Wings' [1936], trans. Chu Yo-sup, in *Modern Korean Short Stories and Plays*, ed. Korean Centre International PEN (Seoul, 1970), pp. 190–219

Yŏm, Sang-sŏp, *Three Generations* [1931, revd 1948], trans. Yu Young-nan, (New York, 2005)

Yoo, Theodore Jun, *The Politics of Gender in Colonial Korea: Education, Labor, and Health, 1910–1945* (Berkeley, CA, 2008)

Yuh, Ji-yeon, *Beyond the Shadow of Camptown: Korean Military Brides in America* (New York, 2002)

Zewen, Leonard G., 'QM Developments in ROK Army', *The Quartermaster Review*, XXXIII/6 (1954), pp. 22–3, 116–22

Acknowledgements

The research for this book was made possible by financial support from the Netherlands Organization for Scientific Research (NWO, VENI grant no. 275-52-002). I am also grateful to the Korea Foundation for awarding me a Fellowship for Field Research, which enabled me to spend three months in Korea in autumn 2003.

The manuscript could never have been completed without the continuous support and help of colleagues within Korean studies, in particular Boudewijn Walraven, Koen de Ceuster, Roald Maliangkay, Remco Breuker, Chi Myŏng-suk, Laurel Kendall and Janice Kim. Willem van der Bijl, Paul E. Black, Eckart Dege, Pieter Dijkhuizen, Leonid Petrov and Clark W. Sorensen generously allowed the reproduction of their images in this book.

Parts of chapters One and Two were previously included in *Korea in the Middle: Korean Studies and Area Studies*, edited by Remco Breuker (Leiden, 2007), and *Consuming Korean Tradition in Early and Late Modernity: Commodification, Tourism and Performance*, edited by Laurel Kendall (Honolulu, HI, 2010). Chapter Three appeared in *Asian Studies Review*, 30 (December 2006), pp. 389–409. These earlier pieces of work were substantially revised for this publication. I am grateful to the anonymous reviewer and Reaktion Books publisher Michael Leaman for meticulous comments on the earlier versions of the manuscript.

I dedicate this book to my mother with apologies for all those moments when I disappeared behind my computer instead of keeping her company. I hope that she finds the result worthy of the sacrifice.

Photo Acknowledgements

The author and the publishers wish to thank the following sources of illustrative material and/or permission to reproduce it:

All images are from the author's collection except: from the collection of Willem van der Bijl: p. 165; courtesy of Paul E. Black: p. 115; courtesy of Eckart Dege: p. 124; courtesy of Pieter Dijkhuizen: p. 150; courtesy of Robert Pemberton: p. 129; courtesy of Leonid Petrov: p. 162; courtesy of Sempio Foods Company: pp. 74, 75; courtesy of Clark W. Sorensen: p. 123; U.S. National Archives and Records Administration, College Park, MD: pp. 83, 94, 98, 109, 110, 111; courtesy of Yi Yun-Sŏn and Kim Tae-gil: p. 125.

Index